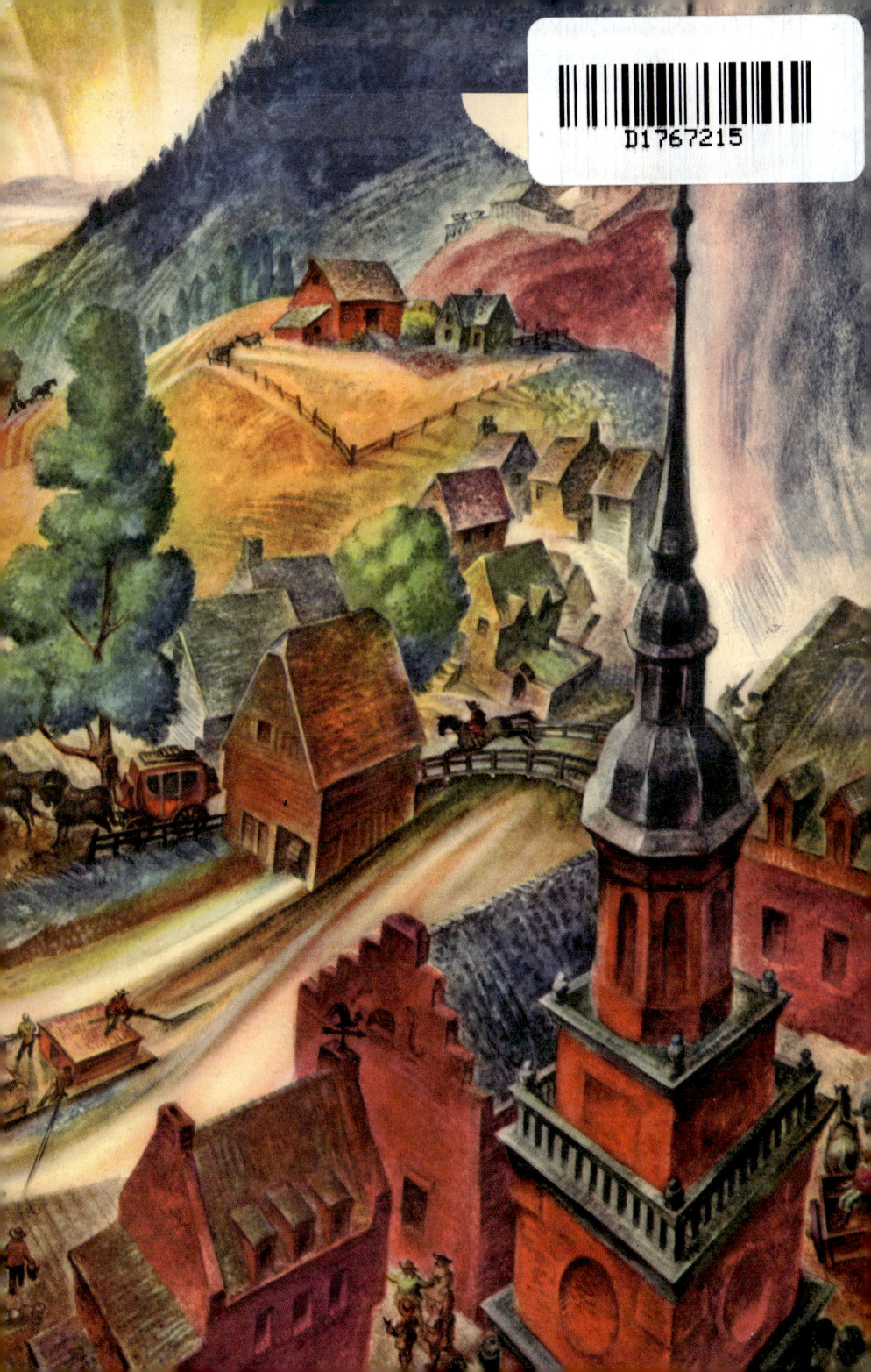

Journey into America

Journey into

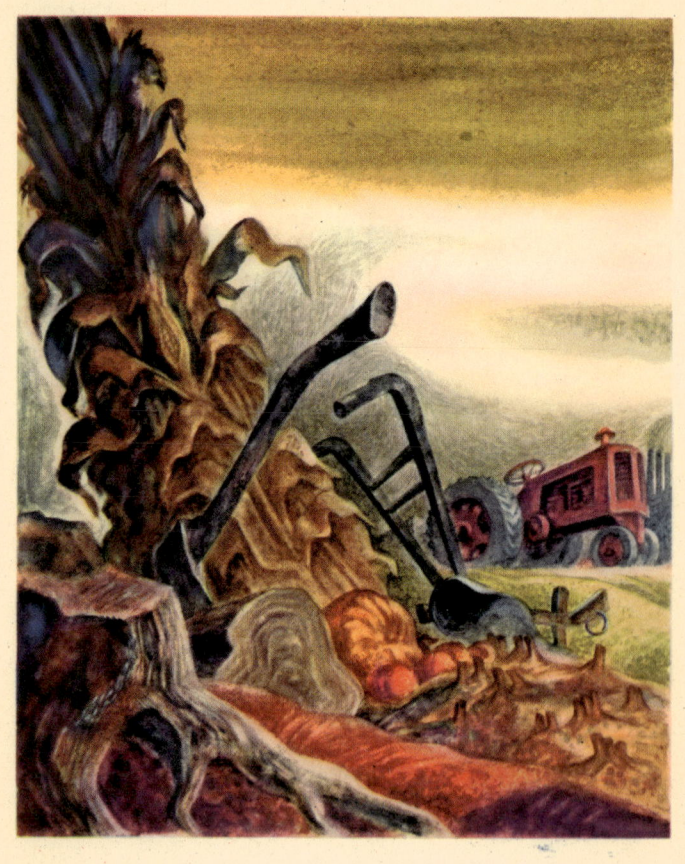

AMERICA

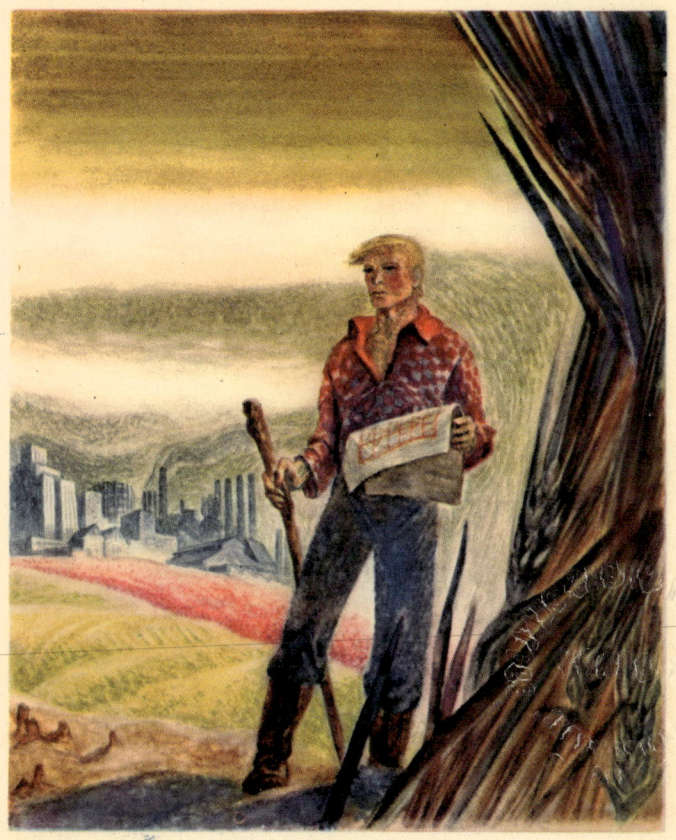

By *DONALD CULROSS PEATTIE*

With Illustrations in Color by Lynd Ward

BOSTON 1943
Houghton Mifflin Company
The Riverside Press Cambridge

COPYRIGHT, 1943, BY DONALD CULROSS PEATTIE

ALL RIGHTS RESERVED INCLUDING THE RIGHT TO REPRODUCE
THIS BOOK OR PARTS THEREOF IN ANY FORM

The Riverside Press
CAMBRIDGE · MASSACHUSETTS
PRINTED IN THE U.S.A.

Acknowledgments

THE AUTHOR gratefully acknowledges permission to quote in this volume from articles that have appeared in the following periodicals: *Audubon Magazine, Better Homes and Gardens, Collier's, The Country Gentleman, The New York Times Magazine, The Reader's Digest, The Rotarian.*

Books by Donald Culross Peattie

AN ALMANAC FOR MODERNS
SINGING IN THE WILDERNESS
GREEN LAURELS
A PRAIRIE GROVE
FLOWERING EARTH
AUDUBON'S AMERICA
THE ROAD OF A NATURALIST
FORWARD THE NATION
JOURNEY INTO AMERICA

Contents

I.	Long Tom Lives to See the Day	3
II.	The Bell	13
III.	The Crisis	21
IV.	Marbleheaders	36
V.	Grandmother of Her Country	48
VI.	'Let Us Raise a Standard'	63
VII.	A Country Gentleman Rides to Office	75
VIII.	'There Was a Man in Our Town'	86
IX.	The Trail to Transylvania	100
X.	Dan Boone's Daughter	111
XI.	Tall Men and Long Knives	125
XII.	Portrait on My Wall	137
XIII.	Utopia on the Wabash	150
XIV.	Jim Bridger and the Bard	168
XV.	Marcus and Narcissa Whitman	188
XVI.	Mr. Carson and the Indians	207
XVII.	Strange Bird Calling	221
XVIII.	'The Great and Durable Question'	237
XIX.	Soldiers in the Streets	254
XX.	'Flag of Stars'	268

Journey into America

1

Long Tom Lives to see the Day

'THE BOOK TO WRITE,' I said to you, rashly taking your knight, 'is the book you are longing to read, and can't find anywhere. And the way to write,' I dared to instruct you — years my senior and by many books my better — 'is to address a man with an intellect you respect, who knows nothing at all about your subject.'

You worried a crooked brow down over your chipped monocle, reached out a paw that had been browned by a Mediterranean sun, and took my queen. I had been talking too much, as usual.

But I stand by my dictum, a dozen years after, and so I am writing this morning to you, Baldur, though you will never read these pages. The chess set which you gave me when you went back to Germany is with me still, set up here in my study, as if you might walk into my California house, as you used to walk without knocking into my Riviera villa, and sit down to play. But you, I think, must be dead. You had dared entirely too much in your native land, and, though you got back to France again, it was your kind that, there too, was handed over to the Gestapo. That is why I hope I never hear anything more about you. Unless you should walk in here, alive and whole with no scars but the dueling swords', that you got so long ago at Freiburg, and announce that you've come for a game of chess.

If I can discover my country to you, a stranger to it, perhaps I shall come to see it whole myself. Not that anyone could take in the geographical extent of it all at once; America is too big, you know. Though, not so long ago, I had a try at just such a skimming look at the land, tracing, mile by mile, farm by farm, town by town, its grand, plain, enduring features.

My westward course began where the nation's began, at tidewater in Virginia. Spring was tender then in the woods around Yorktown, chilly still with the Atlantic's breath that carries by short wave the toll of torpedoed ships. My road ran past Monticello, through the blossoming Shenandoah, and up the Wilderness Trail that Daniel Boone cut. It crossed the prairies and the plains, met the snow, hail, and flood of the Rockies, swung down on the Santa Fé Trail, over the dry smile of the southwestern desert, to the Pacific, plowing blue and curdy.

All the long way home, all across the continent, I'd raise my finger to see which way the wind was blowing. It came steady, the great breath of this nation at war. I heard a thousand voices speaking with one voice, our forthright tongue varied to home dialects, saying always, 'Yea!' I laid my ear to the ground, to listen for what was coming. And I heard that the corn was growing.

I saw the winter wheat growing, too, so fast the Kansas wind whistled in astonishment; the meadowlarks were jingling a pocketful of golden song about it, all along the way. I saw the army mules kicking in Missouri, where they raise them the way the Blue Grass raises its thoroughbreds. I saw the spring lambs skipping and the piglets grunting and sucking, and the cattlemen bringing their fat steers to the railhead at Dodge City, as they've done for twoscore years. Yes, and I saw the forests of this continent, still the greatest timber reserve in the world, from the southern pines, through the hardwoods of the Middle West, to the redwoods of this coast.

I saw the smoke of Ohio factories writing doom on the sky for the Axis. I saw the pumps in the California oil fields, pumping the blood of war right out from under the bed of the Pacific Ocean. I saw the tanks rolling and grumbling back from practice, toward Fort Knox in Kentucky, where lies the biggest gold mine in the world. I saw the wild geese flying low, and the fighter planes flying high, in the same V-for-victory formation.

There's another crop coming along, too, another resource, the greatest. Take the central Appalachians, the section of the country with the highest birth rate. Look at the youngsters there, streaming along the roadside on the way home from school, swinging on the gate, running in the wind, calling down the street. They looked as good to me as my own.

I talked with people all across the land, farmers and clerks and women tending their yards or shops. With little business men frozen out of their trade in cars, typewriters, ice-boxes; they'd keep afloat, they grinned grimly, as long as the American Navy did. I picked up servicemen along the road, men going home for a furlough wedding or on their way back to camp. Hickory-tough young men, kissing Kentucky good-bye — or Illinois, Missouri, Colorado — calling hello to Australia, or Ireland, or anywhere that our flag is leading them. I saw that flag, I remember, in front of an Indian school in Arizona, streaming out straight as if it were painted on the naked sky. I had stopped there, to play with the clean, happy Navajo children. I stopped many times, on that cross-continental trip, for directions, or for a cup of coffee at a hot-dog stand.

Sit on a counter stool there, and you sit at the center of our population. Every time the door opens, letting in a truck driver, a bus passenger, a hitch-hiker, you can see a little farther into this nation. Nobody's a stranger here; everybody is your unknown neighbor. Shove the mustard down the counter; pass the news; ask the way. They'll tell you. They all know. They are all sure of our united direction. Why, you just go straight ahead, right down this road, see? That's right — can't miss it. May be a bad piece here and there, farther on. Tough going in there for a while. But you can get through.

Yes, Baldur, that's the way we think and that's the way we have of talking. We have always believed that you can get through. To the Missouri, to the Rockies, to the Pacific; all that is part of our history — about which you admitted you knew nothing, unless James Fenimore Cooper and Edna Ferber are American history. At Freiburg they didn't teach you any, I suppose because there was so much else to be learned first.

How much you knew, that I hadn't guessed at, I saw in your face the first time I passed you on the street. That powerful, life-bitten face with its look of a likable satyr attracted me in a flash, and you, too, looked into my eyes as we went by one another, going in opposite directions. We wanted to know each other at once. We spent months trying to, in talks as long as our silent chess games.

It was summer, the gorgeous subtropic summer of a Mediterranean town drowsy all day beside its glassy sea where the *tartanes* at anchor scarcely move; the mellow tints of the old houses seemed to melt a little and run together. Only at night the town woke; the lights twinkled yellow in the shadowy pile of dwellings on the promontory, the lighthouse at the mole's end winked with a regular calm like the warm sea's breathing, and in the soft persuasive night air, odors of linden, of lemon verbena, of rose geranium, jasmine, and caper breathed from the gardens of dark and forsaken villas. Then we would stroll for hours and talk, the four of us, I and my wife, you and your Gretel. What can have become of her and her sleepy beauty for which we called her *Dornröschen*?

We talked about troubles now trivial and laughed over jokes I have forgotten; we discussed the art which both of us served and, as more and more the summer's heat and a continent's tension deepened, we talked of the coming crisis of humanity. It appears, in the light of the dozen years past since then, that you were right, and that I, too, was right in my way. You saw things black, and I saw them in sunlight. All that you said would happen to Europe, did happen. But what I hoped then is still a living hope.

You worked all night and slept through the morning; I worked all morning and rested away the blaze and glare of first afternoon. So it was not till the hot light mellowed that we would meet, perhaps bathing down at the little *plage*. Or you would stalk from your swim, up the walled lane to our villa, with your tattered dressing-gown wrapped around your sinewy, bronzed, no longer young body and, refreshed and unabashed, offer to beat me at chess again. There we would sit, in my absurdly magnificent, shabby salon, under the crystal chandelier that dripped from the wedding-cake ceiling, with the closed tall shutters making the room a pool of green light in which our tobacco smoke drifted up and dissolved.

When the dusk came down and the fireflies came out in our ragged garden under the great magnolias and the Chinese fan palms, your owlish mind woke and went hunting.

I never have talked with a man who so often astonished me, left me shaking my head with amusement, amazement, wonder, and disagreement. Perhaps all I could surprise you with was my ignorance, my confidence. There was a lot more that I wanted to make you understand, but over there, in that old town by a classic sea, I couldn't get through to you. But Americans never give up the hope that they can. We are going to get through to you all, Baldur, one of these days, and, dead or alive, you'll be set free.

You can't tell a man about a country unless you make him know its heroes, its bloodied glory of place-names, its stories that are true legend. You complained that my knowledge of Germany was as ragged as your old dressing-gown. Indeed, though I amused you by knowing something about Barbarossa and Paracelsus and Weber, Humboldt and the medieval herbalists of the Rhine Valley, I actually reassured you, that summer of '31, that the German crisis was subsiding! You see, I got the American newspapers; and Hoover had just told

Hindenburg it was all right about that money Germany owed — next month would do, or next year. You talked about a man named Hitler, and I said to my wife, 'That fellow Olden keeps seeing snakes.'

But you yourself had the queerest notions of America — none the less queer because they were derived from evidence we ourselves offered. A rootless, heedless America you could understand, since hedonism and *déraciné* people are cosmopolitan, and that lot was all you saw of us on the Riviera. That I could not explain my country to you was partly because I was weakened by being on the defensive. Our hero then was Charles Lindbergh, and somebody at just about that time rewarded him by stealing and killing his child. Our sage too long had been Calvin Coolidge, and the investment counselor our prophet. In our plethoric era I had left America because I couldn't understand it myself. Was it for this, I asked myself during the boom, that the first of my people came in the seventeenth century, and the last of them in the nineteenth — for this that they fought in the Revolution and the Civil War? The American dream was taught me in the household where I grew up as a child. I had it like a religion, as privately and deeply, but I didn't meet many people of my faith at home. They were there, of course, but what you, Baldur, would have taken to be a temple, by its architecture, in any American town was usually the façade of a bank. Our real wealth lay buried.

So I made a poor job of trying to get through to you the idea of my country. For that's what it is, more than anything else — an idea, an experiment in humanity. So far it is marvelously successful. On how far we can, or will, carry it depends the future of the world.

I will not try again, as once I tried and failed, to explain to you, my vanished friend, that great idea. But I have stories to tell, half to myself as children tell the sagas that are their inner life; and there are men and towns and times I want to talk about, and I should like your mind to keep me company again, casting on mine the shadow of its deeper, darker knowledge.

I suppose there isn't any one thing I could pick out to begin with that is more American than the Fourth of July. You knew about that, at least: that we shot off fireworks and made speeches. So we do, so we do. The children can't wait for the Fourth to come; all along the dusty hot streets of the little towns of the land the popping begins before the Day. So it was with the man that the Fourth most belonged to; he could scarcely wait, that last time, for the Fourth of July to come. To see it dawn was his only remaining wish. Whether he would, Doctor Dunglison could not say. Outside Monticello, in the first coolness of sundown, a thrush began to sing. A beam of golden light slipped past the bed curtains to lay its finger on the lids of Thomas Jefferson dying at eighty-three. So he roused, and thought that the day he had lived for had dawned.

'Doctor — are you still there?' he asked, in the voice of a man in the dark.

'Right here, Mr. Jefferson,' Dunglison assured him.

Jefferson turned his opening eyes, and slowly recognized his old friend. Beyond, his daughter Martha and his grandson Thomas Randolph were smiling at him, through tears — his own or theirs? In a voice surprisingly clear and firm he said to them, 'This is the Fourth of July.'

There was silence. He had never, he realized, heard the Fourth so quiet. Doubt disturbed him. 'This — is — the Fourth?' he queried.

But Dunglison was looking toward the ceiling as he counted the fading pulse. Young Thomas looked away sorrowfully into the western gold. Martha, searching her sleeve for a handkerchief, saw all at once the shadow of defeat creep into her father's eyes. Her trembling lips firmed, and she made herself nod, deceiving him kindly, just as they had told him that all his debts were paid.

And he was comforted. He drew a deep breath, closed his

eyes contentedly, and the sunset light like a smile touched his mouth.

So, I have lived to see the day, thought Long Tom. To see my country weather the first half-century.

For this was July 3, 1826, and just fifty years before, lacking a few hours, had been signed the Declaration of Independence written by young Tom Jefferson. So was born the nation which embodies his faith in his fellow men.

There had been some — never mind who, now — among the Signers, the delegates from the thirteen colonies, assembled in the old State House, who hadn't come there with much of that faith. *We hold these truths to be self-evident, that all men are created free and equal.* It was James Wilson who suggested that thought. What, a poor Scotch immigrant an equal with two Lees of Virginia? The James Wilsons of this world equal with the Carrolls of Carrollton? Dan Boone, unshaven, powder-blackened, holding the Indians off our backs at that very moment, equal to the Adamses in a Boston parlor?

Yes, equal. Just that, with no provisos or qualifications. All men equal. Not only Anglo-Saxon, free, white, American males, with title to a section of land, but all men everywhere.

What a deal of pother there had been over that simple statement! Some lips sneered that it was self-evident no two human beings were alike. Right enough. The Almighty never did create two just alike. But He promised to weigh their souls without favor when king and slave should stand naked before Him on the Judgment Day. Jesus leveled men equal when he gave the essence of all his commandments: *Do unto others as you would that they should do unto you.*

There were some who supposed that he, Tom Jefferson, was promising that happiness would come as soon as we got liberty from George III. Dear Lord bless you, he'd never asserted that we have even a right to happiness — only a hunter's license to pursue that bird through the thorns of mortal existence.

The dying man gave a sigh like a faint chuckle, and lay calm. His relatives tiptoed from the twilit chamber. As night came on, Dunglison settled in an easy-chair across the room, to keep vigil.

The calm deepened. Outside were stars. The lamp on the table burned softly. The long body in the bed lay utterly still. Coma, thought the doctor, watching attentively from his corner. But those still wholly in this world know no true name for the state of one who stands upon the threshold of eternity, looking forth, its peace upon his lifted face. So, before departing, the soul of Jefferson paused, looked back, revisited a day half a century gone by.

Shortly after midnight, when it really was the Fourth at last, Dunglison's patient became agitated. He sat up and began to write in the air, making the motions of excited penmanship. He murmured syllables that the doctor could not understand; for Jefferson was talking to men long dead. Is it now to be liberty, all daring, every man signing, though it should mean he signs the warrant for his arrest and death? Or liberty with cautious qualifications — liberty, if; liberty for some; liberty in the sweet by and by that is never?

They are all aligned, the colonies, except Delaware. One delegate of that state is for and one against signing this Declaration; Rodney, the third, is off fighting the Tories. But just when, in alphabetical order, Connecticut has shouted its thunderous assent, in dashes Rodney, ash-pale, mud-spattered, a wild figure who has galloped two days and all night to cry out now the decisive 'Aye!'

So they pledge their lives, their fortunes, and their sacred honor. And overhead on the roof of the old State House a bell begins to roar. It is the bell on which some prophet at its casting had inscribed 'Proclaim Liberty to All the Land.' The bellow of that challenge rolls out till it sets all the bells of Philadelphia to ringing; the clangor catches from parish to parish, till the last meeting-house of Maine proclaims it over the border to the French Canadians, crossing themselves on their way through the dark woods. Till it peals over the swamps of Georgia and reaches the ears of the Spanish in Florida, so that their hands go troubled to their beards and sword hilts.

Even across the water men heard the din, and they looked in each other's faces. They said, 'What is this freedom that is for *all* men? What is this proposition, that we are created equal? It is not in Plato or Seneca. We cannot find it in the Talmud or the Koran or the Magna Carta. Show us where it is written.'

Here — here where the ink of the Signers' names is still wet upon the parchment.

Thomas Jefferson wrote the words there. And he wrote these, too, Baldur, for all who survive of your kind:

> I shall not die without a hope that light and liberty are on a steady advance. Even should the cloud of barbarism and despotism again obscure the science and liberties of Europe, this country remains to preserve and restore light and liberty to them. In short, the flames kindled on the 4th of July, 1776, have spread over too much of the globe to be extinguished by the feeble engines of despotism; on the contrary, they will consume these and all who work them.

An hour after noon of the Glorious Fourth he died.

2

The Bell

THERE ARE SO MANY sacred objects in Europe that no one European knows even the names or resting places of them all. Most of them are religious. I am solemnly assured by some of my friends from the Franciscan monastery here in my town that certain of such saintly corpses still bleed regularly by the calendar, and others have various therapeutic powers of a miraculous nature. I remember, with tender respect, some of the shrines in the Old World to which women made pilgrimages in the belief that if they left an offering there they would be blessed with children. It is a poor district of Europe that has not got one of these conveniences, or some other bit of hallowed ground. Other venerated relics there commonly have to do with royalty — the crown jewels, the mace, the empty throne. These are not for ordinary mortals to touch; even you and I wouldn't so far violate dead tradition as to rest our weary tourist's legs by sitting down on the throne of the Austrian emperor.

Now in America there are very few of these hallowed objects. That is not due, as you might think, to the brevity of our history, for we have packed into less than five hundred years a fine, exciting lot of adventure and heroes and politics and moral experimentation; we have cut many trails and bloodied many battlefields, and we have produced a goodly number of scientists and a few artists, to be reverent about. Indeed, we are a souvenir-loving people, quite childishly so. I recall that when the great tree in Cambridge, under which George Washington is incorrectly said to have taken command of the American armies, blew down, while I was attending college in that town, it totally disappeared in eighteen hours. That the souvenir hunters removed it in chips does not show so much their reverence for the tree as their enthusiasm for the Revolution, and I am just American enough myself to think that a dead tree might better be parceled out to those who would treasure it (as it appears the True Cross was) than somehow kept mummified, or roped off from touch.

True, there are chairs in this country in which you would not be allowed to sit, but that is because the present incumbents, such as the President or the Chief Justice of the Supreme Court, may want them at any moment. Though there are no crown jewels, as you know, and nothing even corresponding to them over here, there are many places that Americans go to see, either in reverence or curiosity; these we call, not too accurately, our shrines. I shall want to tell you about a few of these, Baldur, though I shall skip a great many that an American reader would expect me to visit with you, and take you to others that will make him shake his head in puzzlement as to why I picked them. But everyone likes to pick his own patron saints and lucky pieces, and I have always believed in writing the shortest, rather than the longest, book into which one's subject will go. You told me once vehemently, 'I hate a long-winded book. A book should be like this!' And you held up your clenched fist.

That was the kind you wrote; the fist that was *Blood and Tears* drove home to me the tragedy of the Nazi conquest of Germany. But when it came out in translation here, we still were preferring to think that Hitler was a 'little' man who wouldn't last, or that responsibility would sober him. I saw that book in a small pile on a bookstore counter, and one customer who paused, drawn by the curiously disagreeable title, lifted the cover to find on the jacket flap what the subject might be, dropped it again and turned away.

Had the book gone, it might have saved you. That was your hope, those last months when the links of letters between us still held. You had a great and terrible story to tell, and it was a new one then. But the American critics were no more awake than the rest of us to what was brewing in Germany for the world. They either did not notice your book or they wondered why you had to take such a gloomy view of things; they winced from the impact of that fist. Later on, when the American foreign correspondents had roused some of us, the critics praised the same sort of book you had written. The American public flocks to buy stories of the Nazi tragedy now, though I never read one I liked better than yours. But you were the first, and the first man in an advancing column is the first to go down.

You thought surely that we would understand and act; you thought that America was always open to new ideas and quick to reward the author of them. So you imagined that, though your books were banned from Germany, your fortunes would be repaired by sales in this country. And with the money that this compassionate and righteous nation was so eagerly going to pay for your blood and tears, you were coming to it.

If we had made it possible for you to come, then I should really be taking you to see my America. Then the four of us would be drinking toasts again, in wine from the sun-bronzed vineyards of Napa County instead of the wine of St. Jeannet. And I should be showing you, not New York and Niagara Falls and other places that the Europeans expect to see when they come here, but a country store in New Salem, Illinois, and a one-story building in Fredericksburg, Virginia, where the author of the Monroe Doctrine first practiced law. Instead of my guiding you through the most foreign and so-called picturesque places in America, like New Orleans, or Chinatown in San Francisco, which it is natural for Americans to enjoy, we would go to a fishing village on Massachusetts rocks and a gold-mining town in Nevada. I could show you the houses and the graves of the New England poets, but I won't, since someone else would surely. Let us two go to see the barns and the children of James Whitcomb Riley's country, and the back fences of Tom Sawyer's town on the banks of that devouring serpent of a river.

But the first place that you and I are going is one on which every American could agree, as the cradle of the nation. It is so well known that most Americans don't go there at all. In this careless class I spent forty-four years. I had supposed, with a laugh, that only tourists visit the Liberty Bell in Independence Hall. God forgive me, time and again when in Philadelphia I literally did not walk across the street to see it.

Then, on the spring day before Bataan fell, there I was standing hat in hand with the rest, to look for the first time in my life at the Bell. In the line of other Americans were negro faces and Jewish faces, the faces of Pennsylvanian Dutch, Armenians, Iowans, Hungarians, Philadelphians, and they all wore a look like the flag hung out in the front of a house. I suppose I'd hung out my own flag, for we smiled at one another. This is the place where we can look our proudest — this Independence Hall in Philadelphia, where both the Declaration and the Constitution were penned and proclaimed.

So there it was! It hung portentous from its beam of solid hand-hewn black walnut, its shattered frame clinging together by a fragile and ever-narrowing isthmus of ancient metal, its great tongue still.

Three guards, heavily armed, never take their eyes off the Bell, day or night. It is mounted on a mahogany truck fitted with roller-bearing steel casters, so that at a touch these two thousand pounds of sacrosanct bronze could be rushed through the door in thirty seconds. Where the Bell would be taken in case of air raid is a secret. But it's no secret that any enemy making a raid on the Atlantic coast would think of Independence Hall as a shining mark, and of the Bell as the core of our belief. For what it says, in letters indelibly blazoned around its crown, is: PROCLAIM LIBERTY THROUGHOUT ALL THE LAND AND UNTO ALL THE INHABITANTS THEREOF.

The choice of that verse from the twenty-fifth chapter of Leviticus was made as early as 1751, a bold prediction as well as a command. The man who selected it has remained too long unnoticed in the shadow of the Bell. He was Isaac Norris, Speaker of the Assembly of the colony of Pennsylvania, master of 'Fairhill,' scholar of Latin, French, Greek, and Hebrew. Step by step he fought for American liberties, defying King, Parliament, and Royal Government, yet did not live to hear his Bell cry aloud the verse he chose for it.

Old Isaac Norris was named chairman of the committee appointed by the Assembly, to get them a bell from Londontown that should be heard far and wide over the roofs of the largest and richest city in America. He placed his order with Lister, the most famous bell-founder of England, for a bell of about two thousand pounds of weight, a bell you could hear if you were deaf — a bell you would have to hear even if you were the stubbornest Tory.

But one would say the times were not yet ripe for liberty, for when the Bell was hung in 1752 it broke at the first stroke of the clapper. Engineers explain that the English founder must have made a mistake in the running of the metal; they tell you that 'cooling strains' develop at the time of hardening, and cannot be detected until the disaster is too late to mend. They say that the flaw is molecular, and that it spreads due to 'breaking down in detail' of the metallic fiber. They cannot tell you why the same founder will turn out perfect and imperfect bells.

The impatient Philadelphians decided not to give Lister another chance. So they allowed Charles Stow, a local bell-caster, and one John Pass, a native of Malta, 'island of bells,' to break the Bell and melt and remould it. The tone of the first bell they produced was wretched, and they were so 'teized,' say the old documents, that they had to melt it up once again and found a third bell. Perhaps all this did the metal no good. But the result was a fine bell, to all sounds and appearances. It was, and is, twelve feet in circumference around the lip and seven feet six inches around the crown; the metal itself is three inches thick at the lip, and the clapper is three feet and two inches long. The over-all weight is about two thousand and eighty pounds.

When for good and all their bell was hung at last, Philadelphia rejoiced. Their new pride was rung, not only to call the Assembly delegates, but on every possible occasion. Soon the neighbors complained of the brazen tumult; architects feared the vibrations would unsettle the graceful little bell tower. But the ringing went on, announcing occasions of joy and sorrow, or summoning the citizens to gather in the public square to hear the news, so that it took the place of a crier, a newspaper, a telephone, telegraph, and radio of today. It spoke to the people and for the people. For there is no musical instrument so democratic as a bell. It is the voice of the majority. Its single tone expresses unison. And the Liberty Bell is the great voice of this people, which no other on earth can shout down or command to be still.

Those noisy days of the Bell's youth were stirring times. From Maine to Georgia the colonies were becoming increasingly aroused by the encroachment of the British Government on their New-World, new-won, hard-bought liberties. So the tongue of the Bell was forever tolling alarum and excursion. It rang when the Assembly in 1757 ordered Mr. Franklin to 'go home' to England and seek redress for American grievances. The Bell was muffled in 1765 as the *Royal Charlotte* came bearing those hated stamps up the Delaware, while a man-of-war protected her with its guns trained on the city. It was muffled again, in mockery, as the crowd buried the stamp papers. When Parliament forbade the colonies to manufacture iron and steel, hats and woolen goods, the Bell roared forth the national rage. It was muffled again, in sympathy, when the port of Boston was closed. Nine months later, its brassy throat brought eight thousand people flocking to the public square to hear how the Redcoats had been routed at Lexington on April 19, 1775. Now, indeed, the great bronze throat might truly 'proclaim Liberty'!

Yet, in strict historical accuracy, the Liberty Bell did not ring on July 4, 1776. Indeed, the motion for independence was unanimously carried on July 2, and though it was a dead secret everybody in Philadelphia immediately heard of it, and listened for the voice above the roofs. The Declaration of Independence was accepted by final vote on July 4, and the document was rushed to the printers. As fast as copies came wet from the press they were distributed, mailed, or sent by special courier. So from far and near a crowd gathered when on July 8 the Declaration was read aloud to the people by Colonel John Nixon in front of Independence Hall, to the tune of cheers, musket shots, fireworks, and a ringing of bells — the voice of the Liberty Bell shouting above them all.

But the big bronze crier was not allowed to rest in its consecrated tower. It stayed just long enough to rejoice in the first anniversary of independence; then, when in September of 1777 it became apparent that the British were going to take Philadelphia, Congress ordered the Bell removed. With infinite trouble it was brought down to the ground, and shoved onto a rickety old army wagon. Thus it began its wild flight, over wretched roads and hills. The wagon broke down and the sacred bell had a bad fall, probably still further injuring the metal. At last it was smuggled to safety at Allentown, and secretly buried under the floor of the Zion Reformed Church. Its fate, had it remained in Independence Hall, can be imagined from the fact that the British turned the Hall into a prison for patriots, which later required bushels of lime to clean out. The Bell might have been melted into a gun turned against American soldiers.

But it was back in place to clang joy for the surrender of Cornwallis. From then on it was seldom still. It rang, muffled, for the death of Washington. It bellowed forth the election of Jefferson. It mourned for the death of Alexander Hamilton, and rejoiced in the visit of Lafayette. On July 4, 1826, while Jefferson and Adams were both dying, it pealed forth the fiftieth anniversary of the Declaration of Independence.

In 1832, the Bell mourned the passing of Charles Carroll of Carrollton, the last living signer of the Declaration. Next it tolled for the death of Lafayette. So a great era in history was passing, passing away. The last veterans of the American Revolution were tottering to their graves; the last signers of the Constitution were dying. And then, in 1835, on July 8, the precise anniversary of the date when it had proclaimed liberty throughout the land, as the Bell was tolling, muffled, for the death of Chief Justice John Marshall — suddenly, it cracked. Never to be heard in this world again.

And never again to be silent. For it is the incarnation of our democracy and as such it is worshiped by the American people. It has traveled more than twenty thousand miles around the country, on exhibition, and has probably been viewed by as many million Americans, each in his day. Little towns through which it was to pass in the night lit great bonfires along the railroad track so that people who watched all night might get one glimpse of it as it rolled slowly by.

For the Liberty Bell is almost a person; it is a personality, irreplaceable and immortal, a hero that was born in our greatest hour, lived through our glorious youth, moved, retreated, advanced, spoke, sang, shouted, fought and fell, in the line of duty, silent after eighty-three years of glory. The Liberty Bell is an American, a great American, like Washington, Jefferson, Lincoln. A plain American, like any of us, like all of us put together. It is the one bell in the country, in the world perhaps, in whose presence every man takes off his hat. It is the Bell for which all the world is listening now.

3

The Crisis

YOU CAN SEE, BALDUR, in a museum in Bremen, the original of a picture known to every American schoolchild. It is by your countryman Emanuel Lutze, born in Gemünd, Württemberg, in 1816, died in Washington, D.C., 1868. This picture is called 'Washington Crossing the Delaware.' I am told that it belongs to the Düsseldorf school of painting, whatever that is; in England, I'm sure, they'd put it in the Tate Gallery, if they hung it at all. Here we hang it in the little red schoolhouse. But it also hangs in the Metropolitan Museum of Art in New York City.

The original over in your country may not be there any more. In the first place, Bremen has been very heavily bombed by the British. In the second, Hitler, he says, is himself an artist, and so, I suppose, not immune to the proverbial jealousies of the profession. And then the ineffable Doctor Goebbels is the chief art critic of the Reich, and he has a political yardstick for judging pictures. If he ever got around to considering Lutze's canvas, he certainly ought to have torn it down.

You may not have heard just what happened when Washington crossed the Delaware. It's a modest stream at Trenton, and in summer you would think that a cow could wade across it. But on the other side Washington surprised, that Christmas night of 1776, an outfit of Germans — Hessian mercenaries, to be exact — and in the elegant language of modern America, he had them over a barrel and licked the pants off them. It was the first victory that Washington ever won in the American Revolution. I have to tell you that the American army, so called, was made up of a lot of farm boys and counting-house clerks who had never before shot anything but a squirrel, and were certainly not accustomed to hunt squirrels who turned square corners and shot back. These squirrels, your Hessians, were veteran and highly disciplined troops, and the fact is that the American militia had run from them on many previous occasions. Their commander, Rall, had defeated Washington in fifteen minutes near New York, by a very elementary military movement of turning a flank.

Those are some of the historical facts. I'm not writing a history of America, for you or anybody else, and don't feel bound to stick to such facts literally, or put them all in. But I'll have to stop and 'tend, for all our sakes, to the picture of Washington crossing the Delaware. This Lutze was a good draughtsman with a lot of admiration for American history, but the truth of it is that he got most of his picture all wrong.

George Washington would never have stood up in a boat that was being bumped by ice floes; in fact, he spoke sharply to Colonel Knox about trimming ship: 'Shift your backsides, Knox, or we'll be upset,' he said.

The American flag, furled against the blizzard, is one of the grandest touches in Lutze's picture. Don't look now, schoolchildren, but the American flag was not thought up at the time of this fateful water journey.

And I'm told that the round-bottomed dinghy or dory in which these patriots are battling their way to the New Jersey shore was not the sort of boat in which the trip was actually made. It seems that Washington's were Durham boats; this is a river boat, formerly in use, something like a barge, and the Marblehead fishermen whom Washington very sensibly called out of the ranks to take his landlubbers across must have thought the craft a poor fresh-water, unseaworthy affair. But what is a howling gale and cutting sleet on the Delaware to the men who fish the Grand Banks of Newfoundland?

Now, Baldur, if this were just another battle, I wouldn't be telling you about it. Even in America, Washington crossing the Delaware is as good for a laugh as Eliza crossing the ice. I know of a better ice battle in the history of Denmark, if we wanted to go in for that sort of thing now, and crossing the Don and the Volga is another story too.

But the hero of that Christmas night was not, for me, Washington nor those fishermen, though I love and respect them all. My hero was a man who followed the same trade as you and I. He was a writer; he was in the army but, though an officer, did not wear a sword. A fighting Quaker, he was ready to lay down his life for his country, but it would have gone against his inner religion to take a life for it. I understand that point of view so well that I am going to have a daub at doing Lutze's picture over again for you, with this man as the principal figure.

I told you that he was a writer; he was also once a corset-maker bold; he was born an Englishman, as most of us were then. You need to know, for purposes of this story, that until this fellow dipped in the ink, George Washington himself was going around saying that if anyone ever heard of him talking about 'independency' and that sort of thing, he might 'set him down as everything that was wicked.' And Benjamin Franklin, his friends observed, saw the argument so delicately balanced that nobody could say for a time which side of the Revolution he was on. Not so my fellow. He had no sooner landed in America from an England which had squeezed him out of it because of his revolutionary doctrines, than he began telling the American colonists that they were, and of a right ought to be, free and independent.

> O! ye that love mankind! Ye that dare oppose, not only the tyranny, but the tyrant, stand forth! Every spot of the Old World is overrun with oppression. Freedom hath been hunted

round the globe.... O! receive the fugitive; and prepare in time an asylum for mankind. We have it in our power to begin the world over again.

That blast of revolution, anonymously published under the deliberate title *Common Sense*, sold in its first three months one hundred and twenty thousand copies, enough to make you and me whistle. Enough, indeed, to have made the author rich — if he had not set aside his half of the proceeds to buy mittens for the American troops, and the nefarious printer made off with the whole.

Common Sense is the direct forerunner of the Declaration of Independence, but Thomas Paine's signature does not appear on the great document which is our birth certificate. Paine was not a delegate from anywhere. What he called himself was 'citizen of the world.' Perhaps he was the first to know that that is what we must all become. But in his time he was just a poor devil of a writer, a free-lance with no salary, a hack working only for himself. Probably the greatest and most poorly paid hack who ever wrote.

This fellow, surely then, you will understand. I admit that I have been deliberately enlisting your sympathy for him, a sympathy not felt, then or now, by everyone in America. Theodore Roosevelt called him 'a filthy little atheist.' If he ever got filthy, Mr. President, it was because he marched in the dust of the retreat across Jersey, and lay in the mud of Princeton. He wasn't 'little,' by any scale or standard, and the trouble with his religion was that he wanted to practice the principles of Jesus Christ, which leads to the stake quicker than anything else. (Your fagot, T. R., is received and duly acknowledged.)

Those who know tell us that there are no atheists in foxholes, and I think there could have been none on our side of the Delaware, as the sun of that cold Christmas Day vanished in a red spark to westward. Now began this crucial night. I think that Tom Paine stood peering across the ice-choked river, his narrowed eyes burning with the cold and their own intensity. He took his hand from the pocket of his greatcoat to dash the water from them. The other hand felt frozen to the sapling where he clung crouched in scanty shelter on the bluff. Those hands were bare and purpled with the weather; officer though he was, he had no gloves. God knew there should have been mittens for every least private. God alone could know why in the armies that fight on His side there is so seldom enough, or that in time. Must it take a despotism, angrily he thought, to feed its soldiers, and keep them shod, and pay them every month in gold that always gets through?

The chatter of his teeth made mocking answer. Upon that other shore, behind those hills penciled by cedars, beyond woods naked and pale against clouds sulking with their unshed snow, there would be fires for fat hands, fat Hessian rumps to warm at. Fires and food and drink and, what can better warm the belly, confidence — there would be plenty of all, over there with Rall's men. But he, who had known only poverty his life long, whose love lay with their baby son in one grave, could think of that plenty without envy. His passionate belief was meat and drink to him, and fire in the blood. Staring through tears of cold, he thought:

So that is the country where we are going to die again, tomorrow. Some of us, perhaps many. At least, we shall for once be advancing. To die only if we must.

The floes, he saw, were coming faster now, faster and thicker. They looked like shunted rams flooding down a black road. If the night of this Christmas Day came cold enough, if the ice jammed and locked, then Von Donop would be over the river here, big guns, green uniforms, slant storm of bayonets. That steel last summer turned the American flank; it would be clean again now, long sated of its revels in the guts of Jersey, Massachusetts, and Virginia boys. Cold sober, it would be ready for another drink. To cross that steel, George Washington led an army that had for weeks been shrinking. Faith itself was falling off, dying as the year died.

A crow called in the twilight. Behind him the snow muffled

steps, but at the snick of cocking guns, he sharply turned. A motley small patrol confronted him; his lips quirked, for these were no more than boys. His smile met no answer in their granite faces, that were alike as cousins'.

'What's news?' He flung them his habitual greeting cheerily, and stepped forth from his sapling covert.

'We're the patrol, sir, for McKonkey's Ferry.'

'And bitter cold patrol work is tonight.'

'Not for Marbleheaders, sir,' was the obdurate proud reply.

'Ah, so you're men of Marblehead!' He surveyed these fishermen in rags of uniform, their eyes sea-blue, sea-gray, salty with doubt of anything not proved up to them. 'A brave breed, they tell me.' It had been Marbleheaders who, with the seamen's skill of their leather palms and the sea's own swell in their bending backs, had got the American army off by boat, when it was trapped on Long Island. By sheer courage, with nails and bolts instead of bullets for their guns, they had held the British at Pell's Point. Now these boys too stood doggedly prepared to carry out their orders. He looked puzzled. 'Well, Corporal, what is it?'

'We're lookin' for a spy, sir. It's feared there's one will cross to warn the Hessians.'

'I've not seen a soul, and I've been reconnoitering our crossing place this hour past.'

But Corporal Nat Griste, son of the Widow Griste in Poor House Land, had been brought up by her to do his duty, and he stood his ground.

'You'd seem to be an officer,' he pointed out in tones that doubted it, 'yet you don't wear a sword, sir.'

'Never have. Matter of principle.' Smiling, he shrugged his shoulders, with independence or perhaps with cold. 'Do you want to see my papers?' His numb fingers awkward with the buttons of his greatcoat, he produced them.

Nat took them and uncrackled them, but returned them shortly, as one who prefers reading character to print. 'Are you a Quaker, sir, that you don't wear arms?'

'I was brought up a Quaker. As for my arms — what is it, boy, that is called mightier than the sword?' His eyes twinkled, as he buttoned up his coat; you could no more impress these lads than the rocks they sprang from.

'You'd better come along of us, sir,' the young corporal briefly said by way of answer. 'To headquarters. You look near stiff with cold.'

Boots squeaking on the snow, the grim patrol fell in around him. It might have been a guard of honor, or he a prisoner. Good lads! he thought; they fetch me in as if I hadn't common sense enough — for all my pamphleteering — to come in out of the cold. A helpless shudder took his chilled body.

'Feeling crimmy, ain't he?' murmured the boy next Nat, and knocked his knees and chattered his teeth in mocking dumbshow. Johnny Brimblecomb had been a cut-tail on the Grand Banks since he was eleven; it took worse weather than this to make a Marbleheader feel what he called 'crimmy.' 'Think he is the spy?'

'Spy, maybe. Quaker for sure.' Nat made them sound alike.

They plodded on through snow, through the cold darkness mastering the day like the despair that crept and seeped through all the ranks on this side of the river. The stoutest heart at Christmastime deserts a war to look homeward. These boys all fixed a longing inward gaze upon a little town that clings like barnacles to rocks besieged by the white-fanged Atlantic.

In Marblehead today it would be no less cold than here upon the Delaware. The drifts would be curled around the high-backed huddled houses, the blown snow shelving up in the crooked lanes. But paths lay tramped from door to door; inside the houses life was warm, the winter life of fishing people, happy because the women had their men and boys home from the Banks. Now in the dusk the lights would bloom out, window after window, till from the cold blue street a homesick ghost could look in on his neighbors all at home. Old Messervey there, bending with long tweezers and a longer patience, was still at that ship he was building in a bottle. Ann Trefry's fingers, between the curtains, twinkled through the thick of her plaits. Mrs. Brimblecomb was lifting the threading spoon to taste her kettle; parson was at prayer, the doctor rolling spills to light his pipe, the very cats and dogs were busy living; and in every house the children sped about like bees that buzzed with Christmas, sweets and toys in their tight hands, quick little bodies tiptoe for to see or smell, faces turned up with eyes in them that shone like the glass bits on the beach.

Yes, that was peace. That was the look of it, and it hurt now to remember. Marbleheaders cry no quarter, never had. But tell us, is our cause not lost? Is there a chance left for us? Is it not too late to win? Too cold, too hard? This new-born liberty — will it be well worth the dying for, or will it die too, like us, in the snow?

For this gray, cold twilight was the hour of our great doubt. We think of Valley Forge as the lowest ebb of American fortunes in the Revolution. There was a deal of suffering at Valley Forge, but by that time we had had a taste of victory, we had a veteran army, and the prospects of foreign help were good. That Christmas Day before Trenton, we had known nothing but defeat, and Washington's army had shrunk to three thousand effectives. Many of his officers were defeatists; two of the most important were as yet undiscovered traitors. Probably a third of the native-born Americans were counter-revolutionaries; we called them Tories then; in the language of modern revolution they were Fifth Columnists. Another third, roughly, didn't know what to think, and hoped chiefly that the war would stay out of their towns and farms; there were isolationists even then, you see. The remainder had to fight not only their neighbors and the Redcoats, who had command of the sea, but the Indians on the western frontier and those Hessian mercenaries feasting across the river.

The situation was so desperate that Washington wrote home that he considered the game just about up. What he needed was ten fresh regiments, and sometimes a regiment a week just leaked away. So, he decided to attack.

The attack was planned for after midnight of this Christmas Day. Its success, of course, depended on secrecy. Now the dark was coming on; the candles must have been lighted in the farmhouse headquarters of General Greene; the hour was that difficult one when, tension daring to relax because it must, the gray shapes of doubt come slipping past even a soldier's guard. One such thought had just been voiced, to the officers gathered in the low room, by a captain with an ironical, rather arrogant face.

'Captain Hamilton's fears are well grounded,' replied Major Wilkinson. 'The curse of this army is spies.'

'As for that,' remarked Alexander Hamilton with dry humor, 'it works both ways.'

Colonel Cadwallader laughed. 'Our own men are good at their bad business,' he agreed. 'Or we'd not know the British are so sure they've won the war they've left us only swinish German throats to cut. Let's not dispraise the spy; he is a necessary evil.'

A quick, quiet maid came in, bearing a tray with a punch bowl on it and clinking glasses. General Greene waved her away, and ordered, 'Mr. Monroe, fill up the goblets, if you will be so good.' As the door closed, he muttered, 'I've come to distrust the very chinks in the chimney bricks.'

'What galls me,' Colonel Glover said, 'is this gossip that Cornwallis is so confident of victory he has ordered his luggage aboard ship at New York. The impudence of that!'

'The Hessians holding Jersey are probably just as sure they'll cross over and have Philadelphia in a week,' said the ironical Hamilton.

Young James Monroe offered a glass of punch, with his lieutenant's deferential bow, to General Greene. 'Then,' he said lightly, 'they'll meet both surprise and disappointment this night.'

As the glasses went round, there was sound of trampling at

the front of the house; a military rap fell on the door, and when Hamilton stepped to open it, a blue-nosed boy stood in the doorway and saluted.

'Corporal Griste reporting, sir. We've brought a man for you to question.'

His prisoner stepped forward. 'What's news? Ah! Hot punch! Corporal, you fetch me here in the nick of time.'

'Tom!' A burst of laughter rolled along the rafters.

'The lads knew a firebrand when they had caught one.'

'By the Lord Harry, you nearly swung for it this time, my boy!' And they clapped him on the cold shoulders.

The Marblehead patrol, dismissed by their commander, Colonel Glover, for dutiful young fools, filed out.

'You look half frozen,' General Greene told his aide. 'A drink of this will put heart in you. God knows,' he added grimly, 'that we all need heart put into us. Only desperation could justify the throw we're going to make.'

Glass in hand, the newcomer stood by the fire, his glance caught by the flames. The eyes of the others were drawn toward him, magnetically. They might slap his back and call him Tom, but he remained an enigma to them. Spare, stalwart, upright, he paused, one booted foot upon the jutting andiron, the fire burning in his glass and in the frosty hollows of lean cheeks. Then he raised his eyes, and there a deeper fire burned.

'The United States of America!' he proposed. 'May they be free forever!'

They say it was Tom Paine who found that title first, who christened our nation. It is a great thing to put a name to greatness.

As he was the man who foresaw and demanded the independence of the colonies, so he was the author of those five fateful words: 'The United States of America.'

That would have been enough, wouldn't it? But that was only incidental in what Tom Paine gave to us, and to those men that night.

And it was a night of touch-and-go. I don't know where the leak was, but there was one. History can name a person called Wall, who dared to be the first to cross the river that night, alone, furtively, a paper bearing warning of the attack buttoned under his coat. Nothing that Paine ever wrote had a more crucial bearing on the nation's fate than those scrawled lines. For on the Hessian side, night brought complacent comfort as it deepened.

'Do you still believe, Major von Dechow, in the myth of an American army?' Rall's good humor grew as he grew drunker; he flung himself back in his chair, slapping his thighs with the joke of it. 'No German has yet seen more of an American's uniform than the seat of his pants. When he has any pants, or a seat left in them!' His head rolled on his shoulders as he collected dutiful laughter from Captain Altenbockum, Captain Schimmelpfennig, and the lieutenants, Kimm, Grothausen, Piel, Wiederhold.

Major von Dechow, standing before his superior urgently, sweated with agitation and with the heat and liquor fumes in here; the Colonel waved him off with a thick noise of scorn.

'No, you are an old woman, Major. Beside ourselves here, there is Von Donop at Bordentaun. And at Prinztaun the English yet.'

'All the same,' insisted the Major, 'if we call in the patrols tonight, and Washington should attack! We have not even fortified our camp.'

'God's will!' The Colonel banged the table in front of him so that the draughtmen jumped upon their board. 'Must I fight dunderheads as well as rebels? Those patrols would be frozen corpses by the morning. Call them in. You may take that for an order, Major. Schimmelpfennig, isn't it your move?'

The gale, as Von Dechow pulled the door open and departed, swept for an instant into this confused hot room. As the light streamed out, snowflakes danced against icy blackness; then the door slammed; Schimmelpfennig moved his piece. The Colonel slumped a little lower, staring at the dizzy board. In the next room soldiers were bawling a rowdy tune; it went stupidly round and round in Rall's head. Among the fellows in there the Englishman was talking loudest, but all the Colonel understood of it was shouts of 'Applejack!' He shook his noodle as if bees were in it. The draughtmen now were jumping of themselves. They skated, he noticed with a drunken surprise, on checkered ice; they blurred like snowflakes melting into darkness.

In the kitchen the black slave opened the back door to a knock. The blizzard, he saw, was showing its teeth now, and snow lay humped upon the shoulders and cap of the man outside. He was eager to enter, his teeth chattering with cold and impatience. But the negro had his orders. He was adamant; he feared the rough tongue of the Hessian officers, should he disturb them, and the flat of their swords. Wall, his stiff members aching, could only crane to look past the slave who blocked his way, into the yellow heat of the kitchen like a man barred out of paradise.

'Well, if you won't let me in to see the officers, you black brute, you, take this to 'em, and you'll see that you should've.' And he gave over to the servant the little paper taken from beneath his coat.

Johann Gottlieb Rall accepted it from the slave in sleepy fingers and unrolled it. *Englisch!* Hen tracks, to him. Scratched, no doubt, by some rich Loyalist who wanted half a regiment of Hessians to guard his miserable barn. Rall stuffed the folded paper in his waistcoat and cavernously yawned.

'Piel — Kimm — ' he muttered. 'I can no more. *Bitte*, your help — '

They took him each by an armpit and hoisted; as they dragged him up the stairs, the two lieutenants each withdrew into a disgusted preoccupation of his own. Young Kimm's was of the innocent far Christmas Day at home, with its dark boughs bearing starry candles, its Minster bells, its soft cries, as cheek touched cheek, of *'Grüss Gott! Grüss Gott!'* — a greeting sweet as kisses. Piel's severely military mind dallied with no such pleasant nonsense. That bit of paper in the snoring Colonel's waistcoat — what should be done about it? Probably it was of no importance. Still — Depositing the torpid Rall upon his bed, he fished the note out and took it downstairs, to the Englishman who could translate it.

But that good fellow now was as far gone as Rall in Christmas cheer. Piel stared at the hasty lines, but could make nothing of them. So up he trudged again and respectfully put the note back where he had got it.

Just as methodic German discipline held, so did American luck. That the slave was obedient, that the Englishman too was drunk, was luck of the purest. The paper that Wall brought might as well have been blank, since no one looked at it with any intelligence or knowledge. It is not enough that words are written. Eyes must read them, ears must hear them, minds must open to receive them. For great words, there must be, above all, great hearts ready.

The Crisis was written by Thomas Paine at that lowest tide of America's hope, in that bitter December of 1776. It was written, they say, upon a drumhead, by the campfires of an army defeated and retreating. An army of farmers and clerks and fishermen, of boys and men who loved peace but justice even more, who came from the hills and the tidewater, from the northwoods and the backwoods, the shores and the docks, the lonely hamlets and the brave new towns — came to be starved, wounded, beaten back, or left for dead. For them Tom Paine wrote. He wrote to answer all their fears, their doubts, the whispers of temptation that promised if you'd knuckle under you would save your neck, your name, your trade — and be a slave. He wrote with the drum between his knees, the taut skin for his desk, and when a thought struck him just right, making his blood surge under his tossed hair, he'd bring his fist down so the drum spoke, a whispered hollow thunder like a far-off cannon-shot that opens battle in the dawn.

Tom Paine wrote as though these Americans, cold, hungry, and outnumbered, were destined by God's will to certain victory because their cause was just. Wrote as though right were unconquerably might. He, who had waked a people so to cry for independence that Jefferson but obeyed them when he wrote its declaration, now gave George Washington a hope in his despair, a great idea.

It was the idea of a peerless leader. It was the order that *The Crisis*, hastily printed up in Philadelphia and rushed as pamphlets to the front, be read aloud, on that cruel Christmas night before the dawn attack on Trenton, to every corporal's guard in the wretched American Army.

So Nat Griste, leaning to the lantern he'd hung on a bough, cleared his throat and lifted his boy's voice over the wind:

' "These are the times," ' he read, ' "that try men's souls. The summer soldier and the sunshine patriot will, in this crisis, shrink from the service of their country, but he that stands it now deserves the love and thanks of men and women." ' Cold hearts warmed; unconsciously men straightened.

' "Tyranny, like hell, is not easily conquered; yet we have this consolation with us, that the harder the conflict, the more glorious the triumph." '

The boy's voice, gaining courage from the words, rang louder. ' "It would be strange indeed if so celestial an article as FREEDOM should not be highly rated." ' And here and there a listener felt a hot gush, from brain to bowels. This was it! the thing for which a man could lightly die, dearer than peace itself, brighter than the warm windows of a town called home.

' "I love a man that can smile in trouble, that can gather strength from distress and grow brave by reflection." ' That was General Washington, done to the life! And Johnny Brimblecomb was grinning with ardor of his own.

' "I thank God I fear not. I see no real cause for fear. I know our situation well, and can see the way out of it." '

Not a man among them was now afraid, or doubtful, or anything but eager for the hour of attack.

Joyfully in the dawn of December 26 the Americans chased Hessians at the bayonet's point, shouting, 'These are the times that try men's souls!' Not an American was killed. James Monroe received the only wound. Colonel Rall, dying, looked up into the compassionate gray-blue eyes of George Washington; he understood too late, and his fumbling fingers found in his pocket the now worthless scrap of paper. But the words of *The Crisis*, served out like grog, were — so said General Washington — 'worth a regiment.'

Benjamin Franklin once declared that where liberty was, there was his home. 'Where liberty is not,' fired back Paine, 'there is mine.' So that is how he came to pen *The Rights of Man*, a book that has never gone out of print from that day to this, a book that caused him to be elected by the town of Calais as its delegate in the French Revolution. Tom didn't speak French, and his friends didn't dare to translate the speeches he made. Was he too fiery an incendiary even for Robespierre? Not at all; he was trying to protect a harmless, stupid little man from dropping his crown and head on the guillotine; he was daring to defend the minority rights of even a king. So they threw him in jail, and he would have gone to the knife himself if Ambassador James Monroe had not saved him.

The Age of Reason was his defense of God, his attack upon the churches. This was unforgiven, in America as in Europe. No one knows now where Tom Paine's bones lie.

Many an American schoolchild's history book does not mention him. It's hard work making a hero out of a scribbler, and he had his faults. He was dangerous — so dangerous that many people are still afraid of him. But I can love a man like that for his very enemies. It is an answer to them all that his fire is still so bright they dread it.

4

Marbleheaders

A EUROPEAN CAN UNDERstand America thoroughly only if he understands one of our small towns. Our distinguished visitors from abroad are entertained on country estates, and shown New York, Boston, Chicago, Washington; they may lecture in our smaller cities, but they seldom see, save from the train windows, our little towns. I doubt if they feel much impulse to get off the train and linger in any of them. From Norway to Italy, from Ireland to Poland, the villages of Europe are beautiful. Time has endowed them, and they have a look of permanence that is deceptive. Americans deeply appreciate the vintage charm of them. No European could be more horrified than we by the murder of Lidice. Far more innocent people died at Rotterdam, but we felt that something intimately holy had been violated when a village was destroyed.

We have villages in America, but we seldom call them that; summer folks from the city may refer to 'the village' which is their source of supplies, but its natives speak of their town. They may call it a little town, in disgust if they are young and want to get away, in affection if they've left it and look back.

Few of the little towns of America would dare to call themselves beautiful. Pretty, perhaps, when the lilacs are leaning out over the gate, or the maple leaves are turning color around the courthouse, or in the snow when the lights come on, or on summer evenings pricked by fireflies. The contented villager will call it a nice town, all right. But everybody knows it took a thousand years or more to put the moss on the village walls of the Old World. Americans have a horror of moss on themselves; they've all been somewhere else, wherever they live.

I once wrote a book about a little Provençal rock town, telling its story through two thousand years. All the life of western Europe down the ages was there, all the mightier movements — Renaissance and Reformation, the spread of Greek culture, the cataclysm of the barbarian invasions — expressed in the daily doings and dealings of one village. Lombard and Gaul and Greek, Saracen, baron and bandit, Caesar and saint, they jostled and warred within the tiny city's ramparts. Its history was, I found, as I plodded through my sources, like one of those multiform carvings on the inside of an olive stone that are made by Italian life-prisoners.

There is so much past in one of your towns, Baldur, that you can't walk without trampling on it, tripping on it, maybe. When you start to write its history, you can begin only where the written records do, and that's at the end of the story, for the beginning lies hidden, sometimes at the back of the cave.

But almost every American town was deliberately founded, not earlier than the seventeenth century, and as often as not great expectations went into the founding. People said, 'Here we will clear the forest and build a settlement that shall be free of the religious intolerance of our old neighbors back where we came from.' Or they said, 'Here we will be poor no longer. This place is destined by Nature to be the crossroads of the new civilization.' We usually know who the enterprising individuals were who erected the first cabins, and we know what was in their heads and hearts at the time. They were good heads, Baldur, and even better hearts. I am prouder of these people than of almost any others in my country. As I look us over, I find that more of the good and great had a small-town beginning than an urban. Indeed, our beginnings as a nation were small-town.

You've read *Main Street*; that's one of our books that gets read over there, for the reason that it's universal. In an English village Main Street is called the High, and in France it may be the Avenue Maréchal Foch. Sinclair Lewis's book is a true report of a Middle-Western town — true as far as it goes. But Main Street is the greatest thoroughfare in America. To a farmer, its lights look brighter than Broadway's to me, and it has this great advantage over Broadway: that on that celebrated and extremely ugly street I might stand forever and never see anyone I knew. On Main Street I know everyone I see, in whatever town I'm walking, because I could speak to anyone and be received with friendliness.

I'm going to tell you about a number of little towns in America, so that you'll see where we, as a people, came from. The American reader might wonder at my selection; he might ask me why I don't talk about Sweetwater, Nebraska, and Concord, Massachusetts? And where is my Minnesota lumber town, and where my Alabama cotton town? If I knew these well, I would tell about them too. I've been through them on the train, and in my car, and even afoot in the days of my student *Wanderjahre*, and I know how much I've missed of them. I'm sorry I haven't got a hundred lives to live for my country and in it. But in the years allotted me I have loved a few little towns so well that I have to talk about them.

I confess I haven't lived in these towns, so I haven't either enemies to settle with or friends to defend in them. My admiration for them is impartial but not impersonal. The only village I ever lived in where I surely have friends and might have enemies, I'm not going to talk about, though I care for it deeply. I owe that North Carolina village my love of our small towns, and such knowledge as I possess of what people say as they come out of church, and what a post office smells like when you're waiting for the window to open, and who's going with whom and kissing her. My mother and father are buried on a hilltop there, and since they were Americans who loved their country to the core, I feel that they have come home.

It was to another village, a northern one, that I went to see my girl, that last spring at Harvard. Not that she was of the town; she had found it out when she needed it and, having known me since I was fifteen, this woman, this girl, knew what I needed, too. I liked city solitude or country solitude; I hadn't got the taste yet of humanity, and she said so. So we went down Pleasant Street, in the shade of the elms, in the scent of Atlantic salt and of June roses, her white skirt fluttering just a little ahead. As we went, she talked to the people she met; she talked over the fence about the roses, and at the doorstep about the brindle cat there, and, when we reached the wharf, about fish and tides with the salted oldsters busy over ropes and nets. True that she wasn't one of them; to a villager, you are either born there or you aren't, and the distinction brands you for life. But who can resist a happy young girl with her devoted in tow? The old women smiled and cut a rose for her; the young women let her see the baby inside the bundle. One old barnacle saw how I looked at her and winked, as one man of the world to another. 'That little un, she's lively, ain't she?' The children seemed to know her from before.

They were a special breed, those children; they could swear like their ancestors (who were famous for it), which is not denying their innocence. They were so simple that three small boys believed it when, at the one-ring country circus, she sent the ice-cream man around to them with cones, allegedly a present from the clown. But then, even the sharp-eyed old men were taken in by a mind-reading act in the sideshow that wouldn't have fooled a city child of ten. I saw one ancient shake his head, marveling, and all the time his hand unconsciously was playing with the rope that hung down along the tentpole behind him, working it into a knot that would have taken both my eyes and all my attention to unravel. The summer sunshine filtered by the canvas was dim and gold and dusty; pitched on meadow grass, the tent was sweet with the hot smell of it, that the wind off open Atlantic sharpened, as it sharpens all living, happy or tragic, in the little town built on the rocks. Perhaps it is that which keeps the edge of Marbleheaders whetted so proudly. There were boys that day who hadn't the dime to get into the tent; they peeped under the canvas flaps instead, and when they were haled forth by a roustabout, they took none of his rough language; their retort floated back tauntingly as they darted from reach: '*You* ain't a Marbleheader!'

When the dusk came down blue and cool, after supper, she and I went out into the town again, down to the ancient part along Little Harbor. Few people in an American village draw their shades; it is a sign of sorrow or shame to them. When they are happily living, they don't care who knows it. And these old houses were set so close to the rocky path that you couldn't help seeing inside. There was Miss Bessom setting a pink-luster teapot carefully back on the shelf among the cups that matched it. There was one neighbor rocking to gossip with another, the cat in her lap — an Orne, maybe, receiving a Glover. There was the Trefry girl fixing her hair, and old Messervey still patiently building that ship he had got in a bottle.

For Marblehead, like a tree that was already tall a hundred and sixty-seven years ago, is just as alive today, and only a little greater of girth. How it ever grew, or got planted in the first place, has mystified its admirers. Out on rocks worried by surf and whipped by gale, Marblehead thrived where you would expect only a barnacle to survive, and neither Atlantic Ocean nor human disaster has been able to pry it off since, in 1629, the first settler, one Dolliber, made himself a house there out of a hogshead for fish.

Just for the good of Boston's soul, I'll mention that Marblehead is the older town. It's only nine years younger than Plymouth. It's near the age of Salem, its close neighbor, but there are ways in which Marblehead is like no other New England town. I'm not speaking of its celebrated dialect which has now disappeared. (It must have been harsh and pithy speech, from what I know of it; it was certainly the most distinctive jargon ever used in America, almost incomprehensible to strangers; perhaps this was because so many of the settlers came from the Channel Islands of Guernsey and Jersey, so that their aboriginal tongue may not have been English.) I am thinking rather of what seems to have gone on in Marblehead souls, from the beginning. For these people, these seventeenth-century New Englanders who chose so hard a home, were not religious, not pious, anyway; their neighbors called them godless. All the world knows that Boston was founded by Puritans who called theirs the Church of Christ, who came here for religious freedom and thereupon practiced the fiercest religious intolerance. (These strictures fall upon my own ancestors, none of whom, I regret to say, were Marbleheaders.)

The people of Marblehead raised their town for a very modern and American reason. They had a living to make, and they made it out of the sea. Most of them were fishermen before they came, or they wouldn't have come there, these Dollibers and Bessoms and Messerveys, these Ornes and Dimonds and Brimblecombs. Those names are among the oldest settlers'; they are found in the roster of Colonel Glover's 'amphibious regiment' that ferried Washington across the Delaware, and already then they were honorable. Up on the Old Burying Hill lie the sea captains in their last berths, narrow ones scooped out of grudging rock; your fingers have to trace half blindly some of the names on the slant headstones, the Gales and Salters, the Strongs and Savorys, the Frosts and Fettyplaces. But half of the greatest seamen are not lying in the thin soil of the old burying ground. There are Roundys and Woodfins and Hoopers and Bartletts aplenty at the bottom of the Atlantic.

These who went down to the sea in ships had bred in them

a spirit of independence that bites like salt in a wound. They didn't take it out in talk. They hadn't the fine turn of phrase of a Virginia gentleman of those liberty-loving times. But they could swear with an originality and a passion that was startling even among seamen. They drank, by their own accounts, what would have foundered a landsman, and kept their feet on reeling decks, and they were as ready to fight Salem or Gloucester, Boston or King George, as they were the pirates.

Now these people sound rude enough, in all conscience, and Salem notes that Marblehead waited for years before it even asked for a church. When the first missionary arrived among them, he got his annual pay in fish, and what progress he made was uphill. But Marblehead was barely touched by the great witchcraft delusion of 1692, in which the judgment of the most intelligent and conscientious people throughout Massachusetts was temporarily unseated. A single accusation was brought in the town, against a very unpopular old woman who seems to have been light-fingered beyond the power of her neighbors to catch her at it.

Eventually Marblehead got churches and schools, and finally to some of its citizens came wealth, with beautiful houses and gentle ways. This honest wealth was wrung out of the sea; the fish from the Banks were run to the West Indies and sold there; and the Marblehead ships brought back molasses and its products, sugar and rum. Colonel Jeremiah Lee, they say, had presently ten thousand pounds to spend on the building of a noble home, which stands today almost in perfection. They seem always to be waiting, those old mansions, to receive guests, so that when you enter it is to meet a smiling dignity centuries old. In the 'King' Hooper house, once more the girl led the way, through the hall and up the wide and splendidly papered stairs, past the drawing-room floor, past the bedchamber floor, up to the empty ballroom where only the shadows of elm leaves danced over the polished boards. There was still another stair to climb, but leading me she paused, with her hand in mine, because a lutestring gown and an old red coat hung on the wall there; the leaf shadows slipped silently, merrily in the summer sunshine over the ballroom floor, and she could not speak or move for a moment, but only laugh into my eyes.

Then we went on up, into the gloom of the attic between the two chimneys of the great house, and higher still, up a corkscrew of steps to the cupola looking out over the trees and the housetops. It was as quiet as time up there. I might have made more of that moment if she had not still been engrossed with eagerly encountered people of the town, ghosts born of the whisper of that old skirt let fall from her questioning fingers.

Miss Bessom's house had a lookout, too; my girl led me past even the reserve of this frail granddaughter of a sea captain, who earned her bread by selling to 'summer people' the treasures her proud and poor neighbors smuggled to her under their shawls — swan-handled teapots and carved walrus tusks, strawberry luster and Spode. Miss Bessom invited us up her three flights — narrow stairs, these — to the pungent gloom of a garret under old timbers, rough-hewn and pegged with wooden pins; dusty sunlight filtered down from a skylight trap in the roof, reached by a little flight of steps.

'That's the scuttle stairs,' said the soft voice from the shadows below, as I climbed to look out. 'In the old days, when the fishing-fleet was out, the women watched from there. Old Darling was the lighthouse-keeper then, I've heard, and when he sighted the fleet coming home from the Banks, he ran up his flag. The first woman who saw that, would come running down the street crying, "Old Darling's flag is going up!" And all the women would climb up to the roofs to watch. For if any ship was missing, the flag went up only halfway. And none of the women could know what ship it was would not come sailing into the harbor. That's why these lookouts are sometimes called "the widow-walks." '

I stood waist-high above the roof, looking over the jumbled housetops to the lighthouse and the giant sea lying level and blue, asleep in the sun. Swallows dipped and flashed across the roofs. In the street below, hidden by leaves, children called and cart wheels rumbled. A fresh wind, old as ocean, came bringing its salt and cold to my lungs. I let that breath out slowly and, closing the trap, climbed down to the two waiting women. It was then I saw that the fifth step, where I had stood, was worn half through.

Probably one ship a year was lost, on the average, with all hands, from the Marblehead fleet. Though Marbleheaders knew every rock and shoal, though they studied winds and waves as Indians the deer, still there were terrible disasters when the women of Marblehead might lose not only their husbands but all their sons as well, for boys went to sea at nine years old. September 18, 1846, was one of the most beautiful days at sea that Marbleheaders had ever seen. The town had thirty-four schooners on the Banks that year. The sun was shining clear, but away to the northward there was a cloud like a thunderhead, and the old salts noticed that the tide was streaming away so that the fishing lines would not touch bottom but stood out straight. Schooners began to hail each other with the old Marblehead password; if you call 'Bodgeo!!' the code answer is 'Molly Waldo!!!' and don't ask me why. Then the hurricane broke. Waves fell upon the schooners that tore every rag of canvas away. Men saw their neighbors' masts flung by the ocean like straws. In a moment many a vessel was on its beam ends, and when the sea at last calmed sullenly, Marblehead had lost ten ships, sixty-five men and boys, of whom forty-three were heads of families.

When the Revolution came boiling up, it didn't take Marbleheaders long to decide where they stood; they dispatched Elbridge Gerry to speak for them, and you can see his signature to the Declaration of Independence, to this day. On the little steep-pitched rocky training-ground, the fishermen learned soldiers' ways from Colonel Glover. Marblehead put five hundred and eighty-four men into the Continental Army, and they fought from Bunker Hill to Saratoga and Yorktown.

Marbleheaders 47

fell into step together, as we have come the rest of the way so far. And those first united steps were ventured on the streets of a little town too — one as old, as brave, as immortal as Marblehead is. The air was soft there, laden with honeysuckle rather than salt; the face of that old town was not rocky but tender to us.

5

Grandmother of Her Country

THE TOWN OF FREDERicksburg is situated in the Dominion of Virginia, pearl in the crown of good Queen Bess, thorn in the side of George III. The first white men to pass that way were Spanish missionaries, in 1571. One hundred and fifty years later the place was an American village, under the Crown, and a half century after that it had become a gracious town, large for the colonies. Here the Rappahannock, born in the Appalachians, stopped tumbling across the Piedmont and met tidewater. So that the ships of those days could sail from England right up to the town. It was all but a seaport, lacking only the gulls. Instead it has swallows, of all birds the most devoted to family life and the ways of peace. To my eyes they epitomize Fredericksburg, as they wheel in the balm above the drowsy roofs, crying their thin, plaintive notes that seem to want to remind the place of the high and often tragic destiny behind it.

All that was still to come, in 1775, and what to your eyes and mine seems a singularly tranquil little town looked like a thronging city to the old lady across the river at Ferry Farm. She crossed over of a Sunday to go to church at St. George's, and sometimes to visit Betty, her married daughter, who had a fine house there. But to have lived over there would have seemed to her as public and cramped as life in a birdcage. She had passed all her days on ample country estates in northern Virginia, and she wasn't in the least afraid, at her time of life, of living alone — if you could call it alone, with all the blacks about.

It was on an April day that her son came down to the farm to break the news to her himself.

He came without his wife, for a wonder, but also without writing either, except for the note he had dispatched this morning by a boy from the Rising Sun Tavern. So he hadn't even stayed with his sister, but had lain last night at a common tavern, not two miles from the old home roof! She set a jaw as firm as his own. That he didn't come directly to face his mother told her plainly enough that he foresaw a tussle between them. She would just remember, she said to herself, the high-minded whippings she'd given him once, and not let him talk her down, about whatever it was that brought him.

But she hurried about her house putting in order things that he wouldn't have seen if they had been out of it. Not that anything was ever far out of place in the house she kept; she probed the cupboards daily to the depth of their souls; not a label might fall from her jellies unnoticed; not even the lavender between the linen could crumble in peace there, but was swept into her palm and replaced by fresh sprigs from the bush; and the door of the cupboard locked, and the key carried away in her basket.

Now she chivied the slave wenches, Old Bet and Little Bet and Lydia, to prepare his room, and a feast for him. Herself, she brought down from the shelf her best red currant preserve, to go with the chickens that Frederick was killing, and the blackberry cordial she made with her own hand each season. Another woman, when all else was ready, would have changed her clothes. His wife, Martha, would have done that, first thing. That was not the way of Mary. These were the kind of clothes George had seen her in all his life, except on Sunday when she wore her carefully saved black silk with the snowy fichu. Instead of dressing, she now stepped outside, to gather flowers because she knew how he loved them.

At Ferry Farm the flowers were the old-fashioned ones, and not many were blooming yet, this early in the year. But she found jonquils sprightly among the green quills of their leaves, and petticoated daffodils, and girl-faced narcissus. Her plain skirt billowing heavily about her in the wind, she stooped and rose and stooped again with a briskness surprising for her years. It was the sort of spring day that they grow in Virginia — drugging warm in the hollows, keen where the wind caught the face, the sky arching bare from rim to rim of the April world. From across the Rappahannock the meadowlarks tossed their jingles, and the birds near at hand called back, unseen in grass that the wind laid about with the flat of its cool blade.

Straightening, Mary Washington thought: the farm is looking its best for him. She gazed away over long straight furrows where the oats were coming up fire-green through the dark of the earth. The peach bloom was just past, and the apple buds not yet open, but the cherry blow was as full of happy confusion as a bride waiting to come down the stairs. Her stern old lips were soft with a smile as she looked at her world. It was a good place, the Ferry Farm, right and honest. The years had woven it into the fiber of her being. She had brought George up here. With Augustine dead at fifty, she'd done her best to be strong as a father for George, as well as all that a mother should be. This time of year he'd been faithfully dosed with the Nines, a spring tonic she made him out of nine different simples, that tasted — so the boy said — nine times worse than any taste in the world. Well, he'd turned out a boy nine times better than any.

She saw a first primrose at her feet, and stooped for it. Not that he was too good, she admitted, with pride in her grudging. There was the mark in the post of his old bed still, where he'd thrown his knife at it. Locked in his room, he'd get down by the big tulip tree; the green of it now was just as young as if the boy had never become man. Old trees, old women feel just the same about some things forever. You didn't stop worrying about a son because he had got his growth. Mary twirled the short stem of the primrose uneasily between thumb and finger, as she took her way back to the house with her posy. What was he up to? You thought, beforehand, that the hardest of motherhood was what lay ahead, and that was only the beginning.

And all of a sudden she gave a short, dry laugh, to think how small, just before he came into this world, George's clothes had looked, warming in front of the fire. She had lain in the great bed gazing at them, sure it was going to be a son, and drawing strength from the sight of his garments, from the promise of manhood that so absurdly they gave her. She didn't think to remember, on this day, the agony of that one, but she always liked to recall what a perfect babe he had been, from his heels to his crown, and the breadth of his chest, and the shape of his head, fuzzy under the blissful hand she passed over it, saying silently to the world: Behold, world, here is the child that you have been waiting for!

Like her own son George, Mary Washington lost her father when she was a child. So she had turned to God as the next most omnipotent being a little girl could look up to. And He spoke to His daughter freely through her heart, telling her what her duty was. And she did it, all her life long, and blessed His name. She brought up her son, not so much on sassafras applied both internally and externally, as on obedience to whatever firm conviction God gives to us. What she hadn't foreseen, what she didn't see yet, as the carriage came rolling up the road, was that, in giving George Washington her own inflexible determination, she had equipped him with the only steel that could turn hers aside. She didn't dream, as he opened the carriage door and stepped out, that the God who revealed to her the wrong and the right might show a different right and wrong to her son. Tiptoe, she reached up to receive his kiss.

Of that meeting there is no record save the fact of it, and the results. But any man born of woman with a will knows at what a heat are welded temper and reverence, in a showdown like that, and there can't be a doubt that they said then to each other such things as they said later to others, which chance has happily recorded and from which I freely borrow.

'This place,' she told him, her head trembling as she struggled for composure, 'has been the very web of my being for thirty-seven years. And now you come and tell me I must leave it and go to live in Fredericksburg!'

'But you can't stay on alone at the farm, Mother. The King's troops may offer violence.'

'And why should the King's troops molest an honest old woman? A loyal subject of His Majesty?' She put it to him with an indignation that accused him.

George Washington shifted his lean giant's weight from one foot to the other, and deep in his deep-set eyes there was a spark, of amusement as well as annoyance. She was sitting bolt upright, as ruffled as a hen turkey, but she still had enough of the old power over him to make him postpone the issue when he answered.

'It's not as though you would be lonely in the house I've ready on Charles Street,' he urged kindly. 'You'll be all but next door to Betty and your grandchildren. You can walk over to Betty's without leaving our land, or crossing a street, right down the path with the box hedges, under the trees for shade.'

He was so right she weakly had recourse to pathos, though she spoke severely. 'My son, your father died in this house.'

Again he controlled exasperation. For years he had concealed from her the loss at which the farm was run.

'Oh, you don't appreciate your old home now,' she told him with a bitter relish. 'You and your lady have Mount Vernon, with its greenhouses and lawns, its maze and its ha-has. But the day will come, George, when you will understand the value of old things, old ways, and know what you've asked me to give up.' She clapped her hands down firmly on her knees. 'Well, I shan't, and that's the end of it.'

So, he would have to break her heart, he saw. And he did it with quiet celerity.

'You must, Madam. That is final. Because I am going to war.'

Now truly had he wrested all her weapons from her hands. She was left an old woman, in terror. Her lips moved to frame the dread syllable, 'War!' But she couldn't speak it. Her widened eyes were fixed on him as he went on.

'I have sworn,' he told her with quiet intensity, 'to equip a regiment at my own expense and march it to the relief of the patriots of New England.'

'Why, George!' she gasped. 'If you do that the King will catch you and hang you on a gibbet!'

He ran his finger thoughtfully inside his stock, lifting his chin in cool pride.

'Somehow,' he said, at once serious and humorous, 'my neck doesn't feel as though it were made for a halter.'

Yes, he said that, and all the righteousness of his cause was in that offhand, American response.

At first she couldn't see it, what George was about. She thought he was simply touched once more by drum fever, which had carried him away, at twenty-one, to the French and Indian wars. 'God will take care of you, George,' she had said then, with wet eyes, and kissed him. And God did take care of him, only to let him get the notion later that he must go off to Lord Dunmore's War. She had implored him then to let the King and the French fight it out without him. And he looked into her soul with those deep-set eyes that knew her so well, and, smiling a little, said, 'You asked God to take care of me once, Madam. Do you think He will forget now?'

So there, of course, he had her — as in the end he always had. She did manage, after all, to crowd herself and the things that were hers into the house on Charles Street.

It stands there still — a shrine today, but no gem of colonial architecture, just a neat frame house like the home that many and many an American has settled his mother in. As you step inside, it smells of old wood and old wallpapers; the odors of green apples and honey must come from the garden out behind. There were four acres of it in Mary's day; it has shrunk, as old things will. Still you can walk between the double rows of box that George Washington planted for his mother. The lavender and cabbage roses and narcissus I suspect she brought herself from the Ferry Farm, for to an old woman slips and cuttings are better than any new plants.

I have reason to know that house rather well. I had been married a few hours before, in a church in the capital, when we walked into the Mary Washington house. First we looked at her parlor, and then went across the hall to see her bedchamber, and presently out into the garden. The swallows were too busy to notice us, and so virginal were the two ancient gentlewomen who then kept Mary's home for the nation that they did not so much as smile when we hesitantly asked if by any happy chance they had a room to let.

That was twenty years ago, and since then the authorities have beautifully restored the upstairs chamber to what it must have been when George Washington came to stay with his mother. Time still faintly blurs the small panes that look down on the garden. The same board in the floor creaks as it used to. It is a stately little room now, for all its low ceiling and depth of quietude. The giant key in the lock is not turned any more; the door stands impersonally open to the nation. All most people would think, standing there reverently, is, 'This is where the Father of his Country took his boots off.' And others do not smile to see on the counterpane a sign that says, 'Please Do Not Touch This Bed.'

When Mary Washington had to leave the Ferry Farm, and crowd the effects and memories of forty years of spacious woman-living into the little house on Charles Street, it seemed to her a mere appanage of her daughter's big estate. In all of a woman's years there is no wrench like leaving the home where she has spent the wealth of her life, where she came as a bride, became a mother, and in her world, a queen. Merely to choose what of her household treasures, with all their associations, she must relegate and desert, and what she will take with her to crowd into the little box they are putting her away in, is hard enough. To become nothing more than 'grandmother, next door,' is to resign crown and scepter. An old lady changes her place of comfort no more easily than an elderly cat.

Clock and bedstead, chest of drawers and pewter, crockery and copper, dressing-glass and walnut writing-desk, blue-and-white china, blue-and-white quilt, spinning-wheel and red leather chairs, old square dining-table, linen and blankets — the best and dearest of her household gear was installed at last, amid the lamentations of the negro women, and the subtle obstructions of embittered old black Frederick. Grimly she drove them before her. The jellies and jams and pickles and cordial all stood on new shelves, in closets locked with new keys to carry in the key basket. Mary Washington then settled herself in her little sitting-room, that fronts on Charles Street, to wait for what would be the end of George's turning the world upside down. Peace and privacy were done with, in this little street-corner house. But whether she looked out into the garden he had planted for her, or into the little outside kitchen there built to her approval, or into the empty 'spare' where his boyhood bed waited for him, she saw her son everywhere. He was always present, and he never came.

But one summer day there was set down at her door a jewel box of a riding-chair, made in Philadelphia to bear Mistress Washington around the streets of Fredericksburg; inside lay a purple cloak with shag lining. It was a peace offering. She shook her head. Not that she was angry with George, she told Betty, but he shouldn't do such extravagant things, in times like these.

She sent the chair to the stable and laid the cloak away in a cupboard, against moths. But often and often she looked at them both, pleased in deepest secrecy beyond all telling.

Martha herself had nothing finer. She hadn't a thing to say against George's wife, overfond though she might be of fine dresses and fashionable coaches. But Martha had never given George a child of his own; for such a misfortune one must not blame a woman, of course. Still, if George had been luckier — if he had had children as well as a wife — would he be off to Boston now, a man hunted by the King and all the King's soldiers and lawyers and hangmen? Again Mary Washington shook her head, heavily this time. Mr. Adams of Boston, she'd been told, had proposed George to the Continental Congress, to lead the insurgents. Mr. Hancock's nose, so they said, was badly out of joint about that. Well, if defy the King those reckless men must, she hadn't a doubt that they'd made a good choice of their leader.

Autumn came, and flamed, and wore away. The grandchildren from Betty's house had worn a path across the grass now, leading right to her cooky jar. Winter came, and rained, and turned to snow. Spring returned, and the old bulbs from the Ferry Farm came up again, hoopskirt daffodils, long-limbed narcissus — the same you see there today.

All that summer of '76, when people were intoxicated with their Declaration of Independence, the power of the King was never broken. George was beaten, she heard, at Long Island; he was beaten at White Plains; he was beaten, that autumn, and driven across Jersey. Every night in her dreams she saw the noose swinging for her son's neck. Right George might be — must be, somehow, for she knew that he had learned what she had taught him — but the power of the King was terrible.

Now the snow was flying again. Somewhere up north there, beaten, retreating, deserted, George was fighting, sleeping on the ground. Even Fredericksburg knew that the game was nearly up, that December, as a cheerless Christmas drew near. Yet all Fredericksburg was heartened when an old lady in a purple cloak lined with shag stepped out of a little gilt riding-chair, and swept into St. George's Church to pray.

She prayed now, not only for her son's safety, for the men that he led, and that they might be returned to their wives and children; she bent her old knees and her stiff old neck, and she prayed, at last, for George's cause.

Christmas came, and went, and the dangerous new year was breaking. A courier dashed through the frosty mud to the door of the house on Charles Street. After him ran men, women, blacks, children, and a bobtail of laggard oldsters, for they knew that the lathered and galloping horse was portentous. The crowd gathered outside the house to wait.

Within, Mary Washington put on her spectacles, broke the red seal of the letter and read the contents.

Outside her neighbors murmured, in rising excitement. She said to herself, My son's cause is theirs, and I have a duty to them.

The front door opened to their eager faces, and as she spoke the frost caught her breath in a little puff like battle smoke.

'George has crossed the Delaware,' announced the grandmother of her country, 'and defeated the King's troops!'

For General Washington was 'George' to his neighbors, just as much as to his mother. He was Fredericksburg's home town boy. Quite a number of them were making good, these days. In fact, this little town gave seven generals and a commodore to the Revolution. Mr. Weedon, who kept the Rising Sun Tavern, was one of the generals, and Mr. Mercer, who had the apothecary shop, held the same rank. And hadn't 'Lighthorse Harry' Lee shinned over the back fences of Fredericksburg with George, in the old days, and married one of the girls that George had wanted? Then there were General Woodford, General Wallace, General Posey the Indian fighter, and George Rogers Clark, who'd gone from this place to the Kentucky wilderness and carried the war to the Mississippi. And, clerking right now in his brother's tailoring shop, and delivering clothes to the gentry, there was a boy named John Paul, not yet *alias* Jones, not yet hoisting the first American flag in history on the mast of the *Bonhomme Richard*.

There is something touching about the scale of greatness in the times of our ancestors. Travelers say it's inconceivable, when you visit the site of Carthage, that so small a place, so toy a harbor, was ever the seat of world power. The circumscription of Athens would be lost in London. Old Philadelphia is swallowed and overtopped by the new, and you mustn't expect, if you go to Marblehead or Fredericksburg, to see impressive dimensions. The splendors of a reconstructed Williamsburg deceive us a little. Queen Elizabeth and some of her successors used crown money to make it the gem of the New Founde Worlde, and Rockefeller millions have given it back to us in all its regal beauty. Marblehead and Fredericksburg didn't belong to royal governors; they were towns of the people, and people have just kept on living in them. Nineteen years after our honeymoon in this town, we came back to it, walked again the same leafy streets and saw the same old negro out in front of Monroe's little one-story brick law office. We fell into talk with him, as we had nineteen years before, and what's more, he knew us; he wasn't even surprised to see us. It was we who were surprised that the town hadn't changed at all. It just looked back at us, with its lovely old quiet face, smiling its April smile, and said to us, 'Well?'

The original houses and trees of this Virginia town are, many of them, still living, but what makes it alive is that the principle of its youth has grown up with the nation. Fredericksburg is not merely an antiquity; it is a people's town still. It is not only abreast of the times, but all the rest of us have to try our best to keep up with the greatness that Fredericksburg knew from the beginning. As you walk down the old street, there comes out to you still some Federal integrity. You might see it in the fanlights or the porticoes of some of the houses, none of them really splendid like the mansions on the James; or, if you are minded a different way, it might come wafting to you with the odor of the boxwood. Bay for reward in Rome or Greece, but for our heroes of America's classic era I say box. It outgrows a great man's lifetime as his deeds do. It endures perennially green, but, more, it so spreads and thickens in an old garden that the hedges and bushes of it have long ago overcome in proportion the man's house itself. So his evergreen glory surpasses far his years on earth.

Box for the man, then, and lavender for the woman who bore him.

She was made of stern stuff, and knew, even after Trenton, that George had not yet won the war. There was no easy road to victory; before that could be had, the land must pour out its blood and its treasure; it must be tested in discouragement and poverty; it must go on bleeding feet. From Saratoga to Savannah, it must starve, and fight, and fight and starve. 'This liberty,' said George with a somber look into the future, 'is going to look easy — when men no longer have to die for it.'

Brandywine, Germantown, Valley Forge. They came, and the cause survived them. But there was nothing any more that Mary Washington could do to help God with her son. So she went on putting up preserves, directing her servants, and grandmothering the Lewis children. She wouldn't get flustered, and she couldn't begin to worry or there would have been no end to it. She pruned her vines and she planted her cuttings and she lifted her tender bulbs when winter came again.

That's how a stranger coming through the back gate found her, they say. One of Betty's small boys conducted him over from Kenmore. 'That's my grandmother, sir,' he said, pointing a finger at the old lady in her linsey-woolsey down on her knees by the garden bed. So the foreign gentleman introduced himself, when she rose to meet him, helping her up by a hand that he kissed. 'The Marquis de La Fayette,' he said.

'Well, I am glad to meet you!' she cried. 'My son George has told me so much about you.'

'And he has told me a great deal about the mother who brought him up!' he said, smiling.

'I can hardly think of you as a general,' she remarked.

'You look no more than a boy to me. As for me, you see an old woman, in her plain clothes. But if you'll step inside we can partake of some blackberry cordial and gingerbread.' And putting down her trowel, she led the way to the back porch.

These are her speeches as tradition reports them, but even history, that statelier dame, stops in her cadenced step to bow low before the crowning moment in the life of the mother of Washington.

For soon after La Fayette's visit the armies, fresh from victory at Yorktown, here in Fredericksburg celebrated the armistice, on November 11, 1781, that was the prelude to final peace. 'The Peace Ball,' as it was called, was held in the Rising Sun Tavern, of which General Weedon was still mine host. It stands today, a tiny seed-husk of revolution. There are four front windows on the ground floor, and three little dormers upstairs; within, on that night, the candles sparkled in their sconces and the floor of the ballroom was polished till it mirrored the gorgeous uniforms of the foreign officers and the brightest gowns of Fredericksburg's ladies.

When they were all gathered — admirals and generals, barons and counts and marquises, Carters and Lees, Moncures and Fitzhughs and the rest— Mary Washington made her entrance, upon the arm of her son George.

'Madam,' said George, when she had settled her skirts in the comfortable big chair at the head of the room, 'I have the honor to present to you Mistress Nelson and Governor Nelson of Virginia.' And the Governor bowed over her hand, while his lady paid gracious respect.

'This is General Wayne, Madam. In the army we called him "Mad Anthony." As you can see, he's still a wildcat.'

'The Count d'Estaing of the Navy of His Majesty Louis Sixteenth, Madam.'

'I present the Admiral, the Count de Grasse.'

'Madam, this is General the Duc de Choisy.'

'Field Marshal Donatin de Vim, my dear.'

'Colonel James Monroe, of course you know; after all, he's

a Fredericksburger. And here are our kinfolk, Colonel Lewis and his daughter — how pretty you look, my child!'

'My dear Baron, don't hide like that behind the ladies! Mother, this is Baron Von Steuben, who came from Germany to help us and whipped our farm boys into the shape of an army.'

Such titles, such glittering orders and bold ribands, such bows from the waist, such uniforms and swords, and names like swords and trumpets! Mary Washington's head would have whirled, if it had been possible to turn it in the slightest. But at ten o'clock she rose to go.

'It's time for sensible old folks to be in bed,' she announced. Instantly that La Fayette boy — she couldn't think of him as anything else — was at her side, and proffering his arm. And he saw her home, through the twinkling night, to the door of the house on Charles Street.

Yet, when she had got into her bed, sleep wouldn't come, after so much excitement. Though there was nothing now, she thought contentedly, to stay awake for, in this world. She heard her clock ticking away whatever should be left of her life, and if she could she wouldn't have held back a moment of it. What a night this had been!

The thought of her death brought into her tired and jumbled mind the plans she had ready for her will. Signed, sealed, and witnessed, that will of Mary Washington's can be read today. The Ferry Farm belonged to George, who would yet come to appreciate old things; also her best bedstead and her blue-and-white quilt and best dressing-glass. Betty was to have her phaeton and bay horse. It was a fortunate daughter-in-law, Hannah, who would get the purple cloth cloak lined with shag. One grandson gets the little riding-chair and two black horses; a second gets half of her crockery ware, eight silver tablespoons, a pair of sheets, and a good deal of furniture. Betty Carter, that darling grandchild, is given the black wench Little Bet 'and her future increase,' together with enough goods to furnish a home of her own. The old lady's clothes are portioned out fairly among the younger women who were to survive her. So, item by item, she planned to parcel away the things of this world, down to her last iron kettle.

That was all settled in her mind, and now she could lie here and think about other things. About George.

Fitfully blew in the sounds of minuets and reels only three squares away in the Rising Sun. But all that barely washed to the shores of her mind. George might go on to better things yet, she thought; she wouldn't wonder; she regarded him as a still youthful and very promising man. But her part in his life was finished; this night, when she had done her best to be a credit to him, was the final crown of all her efforts. She was very tired, and content to die now, in this same 'bed furniture' in which she had been born, and where she had borne her children, the first of them George.

How far down the long avenue of the years lay that surprising agony which gave him to the world! She could not look so far into the past tonight; she was too weary. Only she knew, with a deep throbbing satisfaction like the roll of drums, that her firstborn was taller even than any hope she ever had for him. I used just to pray, she thought with a wrinkle of last amusement, that he'd grow up a man of honor.

Growing by that strict standard of honor she had set him, he overtopped it at last, so that looking up, in wonder, she had seen the skies open and a new light shine.

George was right all along, she said to herself sleepily, and hugged the fact of it, along with the fact of her own mistake.

A last clear thought shone out in her mind. When I was young and he was little, she remembered, I wished that I could make the world good enough for him. Well, nobody can do a thing like that, and it's loving nonsense to talk so. But if you can make your son good enough for the world, she thought, on a burst of pride that swelled almost unendurably in her, then he will make him a world of his own. A better one, perhaps, than you and his father ever dreamed of.

6

'Let Us Raise a Standard'

So ON THE HIGH SEAS there appeared a new flag among the ships of the nations. It had seven red bars and six white ones, with a blue field and a wreath of thirteen stars upon it. It stood, to most people who saw it, for thirteen successful insurgents. To England its existence was a humiliation. Among the other governments of the world, whether or not they loved England much, this symbol of triumphant rebellion was not especially welcome. That was the era of Frederick the Great, and Catherine the Great, and Maria Theresa; it was the time of the Partition of Poland, of the expansion of the British Empire into the corners of the world, of the divine right of kings.

That new flag was appearing in the Mediterranean and the Baltic; it was rounding the Horn and entering the China seas. Its bright flutter was more than a bid for trade, with which the other nations of the world would have to reckon. If the hands that carried that flag ever grew strong, then the balance of power in the world was upset. Many divine rights were upset. Many sacred privileges would look absurd, grow feeble, and at last be tolerated no more.

For that flag was the standard of our idea. As yet there was no government to uphold it. The thirteen states were nothing more than a league of small nations. And yet the American spirit was already alive and challenging. This eager soul had simply been born before its body politic was.

For ten years after the Declaration of Independence our soul burned thus without a body. We had the name of a nation, but we were not yet a nation. We had at last won a most improbable victory, but victory is not enough. It takes a great people to know what to do with a victory when they have won it.

To paraphrase George Washington, 'This union looks easy, now that men no longer have to form it.' But in his day, when Maine was farther from Georgia than Georgia is from Patagonia today, the task of building a loose league of states into a federal government had never been performed before in the world. That sovereign independent states should give up supreme sovereignty and acknowledge their interdependence was a new idea, terrifying to some. This idea, which in its present international implications is still so terrifying to many of us, is the most originally American idea on earth.

Perhaps it took Americans to think it up. For we are a new kind of man in the world. Those of us who came to this country began to be Americans before they got here, or they wouldn't have come in the first place. The Pilgrim Fathers, when they dropped anchor off the coast of New England in 1620, drew up a primitive document for governing themselves; in short, they began to act politically like Americans as soon as they were in sight of shore.

In every settlement, in every colony, men continued to contrive such self-regulation. Their previous experience of European government was not enough to meet the stern conditions of wilderness struggle where rank and family and classical education are leveled by an elemental force. That leveling was the origin of the American form of democracy. The New England town meeting, the Virginia House of Burgesses, are but examples of the great experiment in independent self-rule which our people spent some one hundred and fifty years practicing before they were ready to tell the British King and Parliament to take their hands off.

Puritan and Maryland Catholic, Quaker and Virginian

Episcopalian, had now learned to manage their separate affairs. But they were weak, they were ill-starred, they were foredoomed, unless they could manage their affairs in common.

At that time a wagonload of cabbages coming in from Connecticut to New York City had to pay a tax at the state line. Connecticut and Pennsylvania were on the verge of war over a valley located in New York State. The states had no uniform monetary system; the Continental Army was disbanded; there was no real American navy, no central government at all. The great European powers sent us no ambassadors; where should they send them? To whom present credentials? Although the colonies, through their Continental Congress, had floated bonds to pay for the war, the Congress had no treasury and no authority by which to redeem the bonds. So that the very people who had done the most to pay for liberty were the most thoroughly ruined by the war that won it. The states, through their legislatures, could have redeemed these pledges, but they were dominated by another class of people ruined by the war, namely, the poor. These of necessity constantly passed laws declaring a moratorium on the private debts of the citizenry, and they flooded the country with paper money.

Such was the golden age of states' rights. These rights were everybody's wrongs. So even the shortsighted were driven at last to ask for what the farsighted had dreamed of from the beginning — a convention to draw up the constitution for a federal government.

The invitation to this congress was worded and sent out by Alexander Hamilton to the legislatures of the thirteen states. For Hamilton was a known believer in a strong central government. But the idea of a constitutional convention originated with many men. James Madison of Virginia, James Wilson of Pennsylvania, deserve as much credit as Hamilton, who sent out the invitations, or George Washington, under whose benign prestige the delegates were summoned.

And who told these men to call such a meeting? To know

the answer is to understand how government works in America. The people told them to, one might think, but the people themselves were not positive until the thing was done. It was done on leadership, but leadership that followed popular impulse. The real American leader is the man who knows what the people want before they know how to demand it, or have to.

Indeed, these delegates were not elected by the people; they were chosen by the state legislatures (and sent to Philadelphia usually at their own expense and with instructions which, if followed, would have prevented them from accomplishing anything). Some of those invited did not care to attend. Rhode Island refused to send any delegates. The New Hampshire men did not arrive till near the end of the convention. A few of the delegates attended, it would appear, chiefly to block the formation of a union. Certain of the states were intensely jealous of others. The small states feared the large ones; the southern states felt enmity toward those which looked with disfavor on slavery.

But out of the thirteen came some half a hundred men bent upon doing a thing that never had been done before. Not even Britain ever had any written constitution; its Parliament makes up its constitution as it goes along. There was no path where these men were to beat their way together.

Within the limits of their class, they were a fairly representative lot. There were two Catholics, three Quakers, ten Presbyterians, fifteen Episcopalians, nine Congregationalists, one Methodist, one Huguenot, and fourteen men who had no definite church affiliations. There were, of course, a lot of lawyers, twenty-eight of them, and but one manufacturer, which means only that we were not yet a manufacturing nation. Nine men were planters and landowners; four were doctors; four were merchants or shipowners; six were financiers, and four were public officials. Among them they had had a lot of experience in government; seven had been governors of their states, thirteen had worked on constitutions for their states, twenty-six had served in state legislatures, and forty-one in the Continental Congress, that wartime emergency organization. But these Founding Fathers were not the graybeards you might think them. They were most of them men at the bold height of their vitality, with Washington, one of the eldest, still only in his fifties. A lot of them were in their thirties, several in their twenties. But they were not young firebrands either; Lord Bryce has called them the least revolutionary people in the world.

Now at last, on a late May day in the year 1787, these men are convening to incarnate immortally the American spirit that moves in them. Their meeting-place was the east room of Independence Hall, the very room in which the Declaration of Independence had been signed. In this room, too, George Washington had been given command of the Continental armies; here the American flag had been officially adopted; and here the first Articles of Confederation among the states had been drawn up and agreed upon. Here Congress had received the news of the surrender of Cornwallis, and here had been brought the captured battle flags of the British and Hessian regiments. It is not a big room, Baldur; there is no throne in it, only the chair in which George Washington presided. It is a place without shadows, full of clear light; the sunshine twinkles in the crystal lusters and glows on the fine, plain, white-painted paneling; it shows up how shabby now are the chairs those gentlemen sat in, how old the simple desks. You couldn't have a greater contrast than that between this dignified and pleasant room and the Hall of Mirrors at Versailles where three French monarchs paraded, where Bismarck proclaimed the German Empire, and where the Treaty of Versailles was signed. This birth-chamber of ours is closer to Mary Washington's house on Charles Street than to the Salle des Glaces.

And the men in it, these first republic-makers of our country, are closer to us today than we always remember. My great-great-grandfather could have known them. Though most of them were students of the classics, they had little in common with the republic-makers of Athens and Rome and Venice. That was because they were starting out on the principle of the other great document which had been signed in this room. And they thought about the things that, politically, Americans still think about. How much power ought the President to have? Should the Senate represent the will of the people or, in the wisdom of the individual senator, keep a check on the chief executive? Shall the southern states count the negroes, in obtaining proportional representation, whether or no the blacks may vote? And what power shall the government have to regulate commerce?

See them there, with their queued hair, their knee breeches and buckled shoes. Already the Southerners are talking like Dixie; New Englanders are Yankees already; what we miss is the Westerner, who was still out fighting Indians on the frontier, between shots dashing the Monongahela whiskey from his beard with the back of his hand. He was one of the specters that some of the Founding Fathers feared, he and his independent sort. Listen to the delegates talking, of a fine June day:

Sherman of Connecticut, who had once been a cobbler and yet could say: 'The people should have as little to do as may be about the Government. They lack information and are constantly liable to be misled.'

Gerry of Massachusetts: 'The evils we experience flow from the excess of democracy.' (Was the independence of Marbleheaders too much for their wealthy fellow citizen?)

Gouverneur Morris of Pennsylvania: 'The people never act from reason alone. They are the dupes of those who are smarter.'

Randolph of Virginia: 'The evils under which the United States labors have their origin in the turbulence and follies of democracy.'

Alexander Hamilton of New York: 'The people seldom judge or determine right.'

Mason of Virginia: 'It would be as bad to let the people elect a president as to refer a trial of colors to a blind man.'

This kind of talk opened the convention, was voiced every day for four months, and only died out toward the end when the delegates found themselves doing the opposite of what they said and intended, by making each branch of the government a check on the others and leaving the preponderant power, after all, in the hands of the people.

You see, Baldur, they talked this way about the common people because that was a convention, a prejudice, that they inherited. Just as an Englishman or an American begins any praise of Russia by disavowing communism and all its works, so even a signer of the Declaration of Independence had to repeat the aristocrat's creed once a day or he didn't feel orthodox. These gentlemen were aristocrats in the American, not the English, sense of the word. To a Briton, aristocracy is possible only by inheritance, even the minor peerage not forming part of the British aristocracy. To an American, an aristocrat is a man at the top of his community who deserves to be there.

But everybody in that honest room knew that, in the words of the Declaration, a government derives its just powers from the consent of the governed. Everywhere, from the Grand Banks of Newfoundland to the thickest coverts on the Wilderness Road, the American people were going what they called their own sweet way. (For 'sweet,' read 'tough.') These cultivated gentlemen assembled in Philadelphia were trying to find a formula for safely giving the people the power they already had or would demand. Their fear of mob rule was a sincere one, and had to be overcome by argument.

Almost alone among the delegates James Wilson, chubby, bespectacled, homely but lovable, with a face like one of your old schoolteachers, held out for the people from the beginning. He was a Scotsman, an immigrant, a self-made man, a great lawyer. He thought the people of the United States should elect their own president by voting for him directly. But it's a fact, Baldur, that the American people have never yet been allowed to do this. They give their vote to an elector from their district, but though he is to elect A, still, if his state has a majority of electors for B, he must switch your vote from A to B. And so, the state lines being arbitrary things, it may happen, and it has happened, that one man is the people's choice and another gets into the presidency.

The American reader might think I shouldn't be pointing out this kind of flaw to a foreigner. Lord Bryce has said that we venerate our Constitution as England does its royalty. But the King's a man, and the Constitution is man-made, and the American reader, before he protests at sacrilege, will do well to listen to what Thomas Jefferson had to say:

> Some men look at constitutions with sanctimonious reverence and deem them like the Ark of the Covenant — too sacred to be touched. They ascribe to the men of the preceding age a wisdom more than human, and suppose what they did to be beyond amendment. I knew that age well; I belonged to it, and labored with it. It deserved well of its country. It was very like the present; but without the experience of the present; and forty years of experience in government is worth a century of book reading; and this they would say themselves if they could rise from the dead.

Every article in the Constitution is the result of debate so frank that bitterness was not barred. The end, of course, was compromise each time. And compromise is a word despised by saints and devils alike. Only men like us are able to appreciate its worth.

As the summer days grew warmer, tempers grew hotter. James Madison, sitting at a desk with his back to the presiding Washington and facing the speakers on the floor, must scribble his secretarial notes faster and faster. The first great battle of the Convention came between the small states and the big ones, over the balance of power. Each state, said Paterson of New Jersey, should have one vote. Thus, as in the League of Nations, a small state, if its vote was as good as a great one's, could block the will of the majority. There were protests. 'New Jersey,' Paterson declaimed, 'will never federate on any other plan. She would be swallowed up. I had rather submit to a monarch, to a despot, than such a fate.' Wilson of Pennsylvania, a big state, asked: 'Are not citizens of Pennsylvania equal to those of New Jersey? Does it take one hundred and fifty of the former to balance fifty of the latter?' Sherman of Connecticut, a medium-sized state, mildly proposed a compromise; why not let the lower house have a proportionate representation while giving the states equal votes in the Senate?

This idea, ultimately adopted by the Convention after months in which their neckcloths wilted from debate, was at first regarded as so foolish that Sherman's motion was not even seconded. When everybody was utterly exhausted, the aged Benjamin Franklin was to arise and make Sherman's proposal over again, and receive the credit for deep wisdom.

What Franklin proposed now was to get rid of pestiferous state pride by redrawing state lines so the populations came out equal. There was no second to that motion, either.

Out of Madison's dashing notes we see the delegates day after day arise — the Delaware men always jumping to the attack because their bantam state was in reality so on the defensive, the Pinckneys and Rutledges of South Carolina, very suave, soft-voiced, already transparently certain that their state is on a permanently higher plane than the others. One hundred and thirty-eight times did Sherman of Connecticut in his rasping voice, sawing his hand in the air like a shoemaker drawing a thread through a sole, harangue the assembly. A hundred and nineteen times Gerry of Marblehead — a man so original that, brilliantly right or brilliantly wrong, he seldom found backers — got up to put a question or make objection. Gouverneur Morris, one of the most cultivated and narrow-minded among them, spoke a hundred and seventy-three times, and one hundred and sixty-one times did Madison lay down his pen and rise to defend the Virginia plan, which is essentially the Constitution as we have it today. Anything the octogenarian Doctor Franklin said was received with murmurs of respect and usually passed by as childish. And we mustn't forget the men who listened and pondered, but never spoke, though they voted.

There were whispered conferences out in the hall, where now the Liberty Bell is enshrined. A great deal of business was done in the boarding-houses where the delegates lodged, and at the Indian Queen Tavern. The sessions of the Convention were supposed to be secret; somebody generally had to go along with old Doctor Franklin to Mrs. Bingham's fashionable dinner parties, to stop him if he began to blab wittily all about it. For relaxation George Washington went trout-fishing those days, in the brooks outside of town. The way things were going troubled him deeply. Wherever his sympathies lay he still had sympathies on the other side too; he was a man who could lift compromise to its noblest height. And he had to sit up there in the tall chair all day, listening to suspicion and bickering and resentment. He heard Rufus King of Massachusetts call property 'the primary object of society,' and Butler of South Carolina say that government was instituted for the protection of property. Up jumped Wilson: 'I do not agree that property is the sole or primary object of government. The cultivation and improvement of the human mind is the most noble object... Is this government to be of men or of imaginary beings called states?'

Alexander Hamilton: 'The British Government is the best in the world. Their House of Lords is a most noble institution. Let the American Senate, like them, hold their places for life. Let the Executive also be for life.... The states as states ought to be abolished.... I do not think favorably of a republican form of government.'

In the warm room, where bluebottles bumped against the window-panes, men grumbled, chairs scraped, and papers rustled. The heat grew stickier, patience shorter; attendance flagged. Men would go home for a while to see to a sale of property, or even to fight a duel. All the New York delegates

Let Us Raise a Standard

except Alexander Hamilton quit the Convention in disgust; some others departed too. Perhaps it was a good thing; it threw a scare into the rest. Cried Hamilton: 'It is a miracle that we are now here. It would be madness to trust to future miracles. A strong national government must be established now or it never will be. We should run every risk in trusting to future amendments.'

Mason of Virginia: 'I will leave my bones in Philadelphia, if that is necessary, to obtain a Constitution.'

Gouverneur Morris (shouting): 'This country must be united. If persuasion does not unite it, the sword will.'

In this darkest hour of deadlock, Washington arises, tall among the half a hundred, to make his one speech in all the Convention. 'Perhaps,' he gravely agrees, 'another dreadful conflict is to be sustained.' The warning is one to make all men listen, then and now. But in the face of facts at their grimmest Washington knew how to call up strength not only in himself, but out of the men he led. 'Let us raise a standard,' he appealed, 'to which the wise and honest may repair.'

So, thoroughly honest and sufficiently wise, they hammered out at last the greatest written governmental instrument in the world. It was, after all, very much the original plan — the Virginia plan — which had early been submitted to the Convention. It had been born in the scholarly mind of Madison, put forward as Randolph's, made democratic by Wilson, given literary polish by Gouverneur Morris, and blessed by George Washington. This Constitution gives us not the federal government that we call it — a federation of sovereign states — but a truly national government of the people. Madison explained once and for all the Constitution's philosophy of government of the people, for it was his philosophy: The people are to be protected from their rulers, and the Government is to be protected from the mob.

When it came to a vote, more than a third of the delegates refused to sign the covenant, or had already quit the Convention. Doctor Franklin shook his head a bit, but 'I doubt if we'll ever get a better one,' he said.

Now what was necessary was to get this document ratified by the thirteen states. If nine would agree to it, it was to be binding upon them. The people never had the Constitution politically in their hands, to vote for or against, but the fact is that they liked it better than the men who made it. It looked pretty good to them, by gum. Yes sir, that was all right. They toasted it in whiskey, and they saluted it with spattered fusillades of musket-shot. Why, by God, if the state legislature don't ratify that, we'll march to the capital and show 'em how to!

The document of the Constitution, which reposes in the Library of Congress, is to the American mind the most venerated paper in the possession of the states. When Madison's wife saved it from destruction, she became a national heroine. Yet the Constitution, to an American, is never finished. It is alive and growing, and still his to shape. For the presidency, he has the respect that its stature warrants. And it has been said that it was cut, like a suit of clothes, to fit the giant frame of one man — George Washington.

7

A Country Gentleman Rides to Office

'ONE THING,' HIS WIFE said, biting off an embroidery thread, 'I want you to promise me. And that is that you won't take Billy to New York with us.'

The country gentleman laid down his agricultural journal and took off his spectacles, foreseeing trouble. He looked tired, she saw. Probably his teeth were hurting him. Perhaps he was worried about short crops. And over the money he'd just had to borrow. She suspected as well that he had been grieving for little Patsy's death again. He firmed his mouth now, till he looked like the most famous of his portraits.

'I have no desire to take Billy,' he assured his spouse, 'and no intention of doing so.'

'No, but he'll use his wiles on you. I pray you to be firm with him. You know Billy drinks; no bottle that goes to the kitchen half empty ever comes back. He's so old now he requires others to wait on him. He has a genius, too, for announcing visitors by the wrong name; I think he does it to humble them. We can't have Billy Lee limping about the Federal Mansion!'

'My dear,' the General observed with level justice, 'he got his limp in my service.'

'Yes, while surveying. But not in the war, as he claims. He

told even the Count de Rochambeau that absurd story of saving your life at the battle of Monmouth. But, there, we'll forget it!'

For Martha did not want her husband to remember the war, especially not at night. He tried always to pass the evenings tranquilly, by the fire in this book-lined study that was his favorite retreat. A little wine, a little reading, a little thought, and he was ready to begin his wary stalking of the bird of sleep. So she rose now, with a rustle of silk, and came to stand behind his chair and bend her high-coiffed white head down beside his. 'You will make up your own mind, I know,' she told him, after a manner of wives that is as old as Eve. And she kissed him good night.

George rose ceremoniously, oak-tall in his fifty-sixth year, and, holding the door open for her, he bowed her out with courtly respect. Then he closed the door, looking troubled. She is fearful, he thought, at facing the fierce light of publicity that will beat on us at the head of the nation. She cannot see how she can afford to dress the part she must play. So she puts all her fret on Billy, as just one cross too many.

Billy Lee at that moment was regaling again an audience of fellow slaves with the story of how he got his game leg at Monmouth. How, when General Washington's white gift horse was shot from under him, he, Billy, had dashed through a hail of British lead, galloping up on faithful old Blewskin in the nick of time. So he had saved the general who saved the battle that saved the war that saved the U-nited States of America. Yas*suh!*

His listeners knew the story; they had heard it grow, through the years; they were skillful at leading Billy into further embellishments. They knew, too, that whatever Billy's heroics, real or imaginary, on that day he had furnished the American officers with a roar of laughter. On horseback on a knoll under an oak, he was giving the grooms a lordly imitation of his master, surveying the battle through a telescope. The British, mistaking the group under the trees — thus superbly commanded — for the American staff, sent a round shot crashing through the branches. Billy decamped with his shirt tail flapping.

'I hear,' gibed black Christopher, 'as how General Lee uz so scared that day he run off, lak you did. Is that General Lee any kin of yourn, Billy?'

A snicker ran around the lamplit Mount Vernon kitchen. William Lee puffed like an adder, with indignation.

'*Charles* Lee ain't no kin at all to the Lees of Virginia. We don't even speak to him. Him retreatin' counterary to all orders! Gen'l Washington cotch him!'

'And swore hisself blue,' added Christopher.

This legend of Washington's profanity always enraged Billy.

"Twas me cussed,' he cried, on a sudden improvisation. 'I cussed fo' His Excellency, 'cause he cain't rightly do it. I cussed twell the leaves blush red like Octobah and fall off the trees. I cussed twell the calvary hawses done faint. I cussed twell Gen'l Lee turn round and face the Briddish, to get away from my cussin'!'

A high African cackle of glee, mingling derision and delight, rose to the beams. Then a bell sounded sharply rung in the master's study.

'No, Billy,' the General was telling him a few minutes later, 'I can't take you to New York. That's final.' He put his palm down so sharply on the little table that the Madeira Billy had just poured leaped in its goblet.

'Yassuh, co'se it's final,' Billy agreed cheerfully. 'Cain't be no othah way, when a body ain't made up they min' yit.'

Washington sipped his glass; the Madeira gave its little mellow dig at his vitals, and heartened his patience.

'You see, Billy,' he began, 'New York's a mighty fashionable place. Now that it's to be the temporary capital of our country, it will be twice as strict in its social observances. And the Federal Mansion will be the place on which all eyes will be fixed. Here in the country we live simply. Up with the birds, to go fox-hunting or ride over the farms. And early to bed, no matter who the guests are.'

'Yassuh,' Billy nodded. 'Mighty peaceful and sleepy. Don't no-ways use our talents.'

Washington suppressed a smile. 'In New York we'll be like soldiers in dress-parade uniform all the time, standing at attention, before all those ambassadors and statesmen and great ladies.' He closed his eyes in weariness at the thought, and so missed the expression of charmed anticipation that broke over Billy's old face. 'I don't know,' the General murmured, 'how at my age I am going to stand it.' Or afford it, he added in thought.

'I reckon I see now,' Billy singsonged with dark racial melancholy. 'Ain't no place for pore ol' Billy now we's president. Him and Blewskin gotta turn out to grass till they bones falls apaht. Time was when the sight of 'em were mighty good!'

But Billy, the General decided, couldn't trade on Monmouth again.

'Laws amassy, it were hot at Monmuff! Whee-*yew!*' Billy mopped his brow, and experimentally slipped the chisel in elsewhere. 'Hot at Monmuff as it were col' at Valley Fawge!'

The two words rang through the room like bells of ice. The carpet became a drift of dirty snow, with blood on it from soldiers' feet. The log on the hearth fell; in the tense quiet Billy observed his master silent in reminiscence, and stood breathing carefully, to efface himself. To Washington, the log had become the butt of a musket burning to warm frozen hands back to pain. Unconsciously the General pushed the Madeira aside, like a comfort out of place. The book-lined walls of the room were logs of his cabin; the wind and snow sailed through the cracks of them. The agricultural journal on his knee was that insulting, whining, obstructive note from Congress, telling why it could not send money to pay the men — though Congress drew its own pay. And why those well-shod, well-fed, and soundly sleeping gentlemen could not provide shoes nor blankets, nor food nor ammunition. Washington closed his eyes. One morning, the coldest of all, when he had opened them, it had been to see Billy's coat laid over his sleeping body, with the blown snow caught in the threadbare folds. Those eyes opened now, looking from far away at the bent old slave.

'So you're determined to come, Billy? Well, I can't deny you. I shall be glad, indeed,' he made himself kindly say, 'if you keep sober and show proper respect to your mistress, to keep you beside me.'

Some days ahead of his master — by Washington's own old account book — Billy left, in company with Colonel Tobias Lear, factotum of the estate of Mount Vernon. He was in his glory, clad in the newly ordered livery of the estate — blue broadcloth trimmed with silver lace. He was perhaps high with wine as well as pride as he limped across to Chinkling whom he had ridden so long, as master of hounds, the silver horn at his shoulder. But his attempts to get into the saddle only showed how far gone he was in age. Two sniggering stable boys had to boost him to the back of the reproachful Chinkling, who looked around in disgust. Once in the saddle Billy doffed his cap magnificently, showing his kinky white curls.

'You needn' to worry 'bout a thing,' he told his master grandly. 'Billy goin' on ahead to Noo Yawk to open up the Federal Mansion! Depen' on him. He'll always be right on han'!'

And right under foot, thought Washington dubiously, as he waved his hand in farewell.

In the crowded days that followed, Billy was forgotten except for ominous references to his decline in Lear's letters. His master had heavier cares. Not the least of his regrets was at missing the spring that never stole up the land more sweetly than in the year that the master of Mount Vernon left it. Spring took the world with plum-blow at the Dogue Run Farm, with redbud in the 'Wilderness' behind the 'home house,' as Washington called Mount Vernon mansion. She was piped in, at Union Farm, by the peepers. The redwings welcomed her, over at the River Farm, with jingling cries. At Muddy Hole Farm she was greeted with bleats; these were the finest lambings the master had ever seen.

As he rode his lands each day, he knew he had never loved them more. He loved the Dogue Run Farm for its thundering grist mill, with its mossy overshot wheel and the sixteen-sided barns and the creaking ferry, the old ferryman and the fine fishing. Muddy Hole ran at a loss, in itself, but, rudest of them all, it paid its way in the black muck and the sheep dung that it yielded to the other fields. Washington had a modern farmer's understanding of good fertilizer, and a respect for it.

The Mansion Farm he loved for its box hedges and the lawns where the children rolled, and above all for the trees that he had planted. There were lindens sent by Governor Clinton of New York, and hemlocks brought from the Blue Ridge. Twelve horsechestnuts given by 'Lighthorse Harry' Lee grew there, and a row of cypresses presented by the King of France; live-oaks had years ago been brought from the Tidewater down Norfolk way and, from the savage Ohio frontier, buckeyes and Kentucky coffee-trees. He loved the English mulberries he had grafted on the wild ones, and the grafts he'd made of apple and pear on quince. And the bullock-heart and coronation cherries just now budding out on the smooth red wood. He loved the home house because it was the core of all his being. Here six babies had been born. Here six men and women were buried, last of them his beloved Patsy, his stepdaughter-sweetheart, Miss Martha Parke Custis, dead in her seventeenth year and mourned by him every day of his life.

He loved the River Farm because it grew the finest wheat. True, it did not really pay. But when did farming ever pay? One year it was drought — like 1785 — when the wheat fired in the ear, and chinch bugs were a plague of Egypt. Next, as in 1786, the disaster was flood, and they read the prayer

For Fair Weather every Sunday in Pohick church. When the wheat crop was good, the price fell; when the price rose, that was because of short crops. And because of short crops he had had to go with his hat in his hand and borrow money at interest, in order to shoulder the expenses of the presidency.

But a farmer is paid in his way of life. G. Washington, Esquire, was born to that way, born to be a wheat farmer. So he had chosen to add heads of wheat to the stars and bars of the Washington coat-of-arms, when he designed his bookplate. He grew wheat when everyone told him that a Virginia farmer could only make money by sticking to the one-crop system — tobacco, the state's only export. What if it did exhaust the soil? Abandon the farm, cut down new woods, use up the thin humus, and move on again, they said with a shrug. This was a mighty big new country.

But George Washington was a faithful husbandman to his acres. He built them up, with careful study in his books, and wrote to Arthur Young in England about fertilizers. Farming by correspondence! his neighbors chuckled. They laughed at his drill plow that he invented and was always improving. They laughed at the roller he used to press the seeds down in the furrow. They laughed because he sowed earlier than they, and cut when the crop was green. Not tobacco but wheat — green in the leaf, gold in the ear, white in the loaf. Good wheat, sown from the best seed. 'The best comes from the best,' said G. Washington, Esquire.

Yet even those wheatfields had tares in them.

'*When the blade was sprung up and brought forth fruit, then appeared the tares also.*' The minister at Pohick read out the text from Matthew. In his pew George Washington bowed his head. Tares in the field, in every man's soul, and in every nation.

The day of departure came in one stride. His wife and the grandchildren were to follow. Now in the 'white chariot,' the big coach with cream-colored body and wheels and the Washington arms on the door, the country gentleman drew on his lemon-colored gloves, as he seated himself beside his secretary, Colonel Humphrey, and old Thompson, the Secretary of Congress. Washington signed to the driver to roll on. In a moment the home house had vanished.

These are the things, which once possess'd — he quoted with silent, moving lips, from a poem he had got by heart in boyhood — *will make a life that's truly bless'd. A good estate, a healthy soul* —

'I beg your pardon, sir?' said Colonel Humphrey politely.

Washington smiled. 'Nothing, Colonel,' he said. 'A bit of doggerel, that's all.'

But the lines ran after him wistfully:

> Round a warm fire, a pleasant joke.
> A chimney ever free from smoke —

The 'Wilderness' was flashing by. Little crimson keys were on the maples. How beautiful they looked, contrasted with the pale honey-colored flowers of sassafras! All the freshness of the April day assailed him and his five senses, like beguiling children, reproached him for leaving. Carolina wrens whistled after the bowling coach, inviting him, if he must go somewhere, to ride these woods for foxes. The fragrant azalea and the bloodroot asked him what would he find fairer? As the carriage swung out on the last of his fields, the odor of turned earth rose from the furrows and called and called him back.

'Stop!' Washington called to the coachman. 'Stop here!'

Swinging open the carriage door, he brushed angrily past old Thompson's knees and went leaping across the ground with a wiry agility.

The overseer beating the cringing negro about the head did not see his employer until Washington sprang on him. Colonel Humphrey leaped from the carriage to come to the aid of the President. But Washington had wrenched the stick free in a single twist; the overseer staggered back, and as Washington lifted the rod, he backed away, covering his face.

'Remember your character, Mr. Washington. For God's sake, remember your character!'

Lowering his arm, George Washington remembered it, and chucked the stick to the ground. Then he spoke, and his voice fell like a blow.

'If you must beat a man, a slave or a soldier, you may beat his back — if you know you're right and he will learn in no other way. But not a man's face and head, you scoundrel!'

He turned and started to stride away. Then he walked back; ignorance deserved a more patient lesson.

'God never made the man to whom He didn't give human dignity the equal of any other man's,' he quietly said. 'Unless it's an overseer. You may go to the house and receive your pay. You're finished here.'

Then he stooped and raised the young negro up. With his handkerchief he wiped the blood from the man's face, revealing bronze Ashanti features. His master realized with distress that he did not even recognize him. There were forty slaves on the Dogue Run Farm, and fifty on the Union Farm, thirty at Muddy Hole and sixty at the River Farm — almost two hundred, counting the house and stable servants.

'Who are you?' he demanded kindly.

'I'se Tobie,' said the slave humbly. 'Polly Cottah's boy.'

'Go home to her, Tobie, and tell her to send for the mistress to poultice that face of yours. Go along now, and God forgive us!' he muttered.

Within the coach, as it rumbled on, there was oppressive silence. Mr. Thompson felt as guilty as the overseer, he did not know why, and Humphrey's face was downcast. A lightning bolt stripping the bark of a tree beside them couldn't have sizzled the air more fiercely. They could well believe that General Washington had not cursed Lee at Monmouth. He wouldn't require swear-words. His terrible, leashed anger could curse a man for life, as it had blasted Lee out of the war.

Locked in himself, Washington had forgotten his anger with the overseer. That sterilizing wrath was turned upon himself, and the rest of his fields rolled past his averted eyes. For slavery was the tares in the land that he could not bear to look upon.

This black institution he had inherited, both as a property-owner and as the nation's first President. Years ago he had made the resolve never to buy another human being, but they came on, like Tobie out of Polly, slave children in a dark and rising flood. The tares were thorny to the hand; they were growing to the sky, until the trees said to the brambles, *Come and reign over us.* A Devil's curse. And like so many of the Devil's bargains, it paid out handsomely, at first. It paid in ease and pride and comforts of the flesh. But the price was yet to be demanded.

That in his will he freed his own slaves was nothing, he knew, but a sop to his individual conscience. Yet it was all that he saw to do. Even at the Constitutional Convention, the very men who declared it to be self-evident that all men are born free and equal had not been able to uproot these weeds.

So the servants of the householder came and said to him, *Wilt thou then that we go and gather them up? But he said, Nay: lest while ye gather up the tares, ye root up also the wheat with them.*

Madison, Wilson, Hamilton, old Ben Franklin, and other wise men who hammered out the Constitution, through the long hot months of summer — they had seen, as the householder saw, that to tear out slavery from the young nation they were creating would have torn up the nation itself by the roots. So they had sown the tares with the wheat, when they signed the great document. So, too, Washington felt on his bowed shoulders an obligation to all his black brothers. Not for Monmouth or Valley Forge, but for this, he had given old Billy Lee his faithful heart's desire.

Yet a hand stronger and gentler than George Washington's own put this decision aside. In Philadelphia, when he arrived there, he found Billy Lee flat on his back in bed.

'I nevah fail you befo', Gen'l,' quavered the weak old voice, and a hand like a monkey's ventured a worshipful clutch at his sleeve. 'But I'se plumb tuckud. I'se too ol' fo' you now, Gen'l. The Lawd, He showed me. He humble me. I uz too proud.'

A Country Gentleman Rides to Office 85

The tall man standing above him stooped for a firm caress of his shoulder. 'That's all right, Billy. We are all too proud, perhaps. You want to go home now, don't you?' He straightened; the tired slave nodded, glad peace in his face. 'So do I, Billy,' the General murmured. 'So do I!'

But ahead lay a new, an unprecedented duty. Ahead lay the bunting and fireworks, the cheers and the crowds and the speeches, of the first inaugural of the first President of the United States of America. Beyond all that temporal glory lay the future of the newly created nation. Now the farmer-statesman saw this people, sown in the furrows of the Revolution, sprung up like wheat, green in the leaf. He foresaw a golden harvest, reaching in time from sea to sea, but having, in time, no limit. And he saw that the wheat had tares in it.

Standing at his slave's bedside, the President-Elect himself felt humbled. The old negro, he noticed, had fallen asleep. Black and white, we must go on together; for all the faults in it, the nation must march forward. But the time must come, he thought strongly, when we shall uproot those evils, root, stem, and branch. Not negro slavery only, but all the other slaveries into which men sell themselves; the power of money, the lust of power, the sloth that comes with having, the hatred come of not having enough. In the time of harvest I will say to the reapers, *Gather ye together first the tares, and bind them in bundles to burn them.* Hands stronger than mine, unborn, shall uproot them, George Washington said to himself, staring into America's future. Not until then will the freedom I fought for be granted Americans!

8

'There Was a Man in Our Town'

WE DARE TO BE SO intimate, Baldur, with even our greatest national heroes because they are none of them set apart from us, nor ever were. The British, who have come to love their king almost fraternally, still are proud of that crown of his. Headgear has been pretty much the same for all of us over here, sometimes a cocked hat, sometimes a stovepipe, and nobody but his wife was much upset when the President-Elect, at a knock on the door of his Springfield house, used to go to open it himself in his old slippers. We see our great men simply as men like us, only far better, and we don't love or venerate them the less for that. The mother of any boy born in this country can, and usually does, think at some time or other that he might grow up to be President of the United States; a rare exception among our mothers must have been Mary Ball Washington.

What makes us feel so close to the Founding Fathers is that we believe as they did. However much our circumstances have changed and our ways and means have broadened and quickened, we are still as a nation doing business on the same old stand which they took up. Sometimes some of us get to doubting this, and when a man does, he's unhappy. We are afraid to get any distance away from the beginning they made for us, which was so risky and unprecedented then, and now looks like the only safety. And, of course, we have got as far from that beginning as a young man has got from the baby he was when he lay in his cradle. There's no harm in sentiment about the old family cradle, but it is very dangerous for a youth to decline to grow up.

I want you to meet some of my friends of today, Baldur, as well as the men of yesterday, even if you catch a few of us having the cramps of growing pains. For the Americans you knew in Europe were an exceptional lot, or they wouldn't have been there. The great majority of my people have never been to Europe and don't plan to go. This is not due to pride; I'd almost say it was a sign of humility. It is startling to find that one's views and almost one's person are treated with a certain respect, in provincial places, if it's discovered that one has lived in foreign countries. Indeed, if I wanted to gain the confidence of an Arizona ranchman, and have him talk to me at his ease, I'd hold back the fact of knowing you and loving you, of living for years on the Riviera, and even of having gone to an eastern college. All these facts would arouse no hostility in what is probably the fairest and most friendly kind of man in the world; but such disclosures might drive him into taciturnity. The world over, I suppose, a man is his best on home ground.

I recall a conversation I made once with an Indiana farmer, where I stopped on a tramp for a drink from his well. 'Mighty pretty place you've got here,' I remarked, gazing down through his woods to the ferny limestone dell.

'Yes,' he admitted, 'some of the prettiest places in the world are right around here.'

I emptied his glass of well water, thanked him and departed smiling to myself. Poor fellow, I thought, he hasn't seen much! I was a youngster and fed up — for life, I supposed — with his kind of scenery. Hadn't I been to New England and western North Carolina, Scotland, Devon, and Normandy? And wouldn't I jump at the chance to see the Alps, the Mediterranean, the famous and spectacular beauties of the Côte d'Azur?

I got the chance, and took it, and all I saw was as advertised. I loved it, and thought I was at home there, till there came those hard times that test the friendliness in places. Then it was really home I wanted, and when an American says home, he is not apt to mean Niagara Falls or the rim of the Grand Canyon or the top of Pike's Peak or any of the other natural grandeurs by which those who have never seen this country may try to visualize it. No, it wasn't postal-card scenery that I remembered with an ache. I was longing for those islands, moored like steamboats, in our big rivers, and the dreamy, vine-clad woods that they carry. It was little thorn apples in autumn I wanted, shining like Christmas trees with their freight of tart, rosy haws. It was bobolink song in a meadow dancing with Queen Anne's lace, and the way crow calls come to you over a still, cold lake in Wisconsin northwoods.

That first attack of homesickness was my last, for it was a lasting one. Coming home did not cure me. I have spent much of my time and money since in trying to slake an unquenchable thirst for this land of ours, and I still think that if ever you can catch a glimpse of the soul of all America, it is in the dusk, framed by a Pullman window, where the first lights gleam in vanishing little towns, in lonely farms, in lost cabins, where the waiter goes past you chanting, 'Dinah in the reah! Fust call...' and the engine 'way up ahead cries *Woooooooo! woo-woo!* as it plunges into the big swamp woods and the thickening night. Beyond the dark window where reflections of your own face hide a continent, lie the thousand fragments of our great whole, which are home to a people.

The results of a mild but chronic case of *nostalgia americana* like mine are that the more you go round, the more places you have to miss, when the trains whistle. But the man who has not traveled far puts all his heart into the scenes with which he has been familiar always. Most of the men in uniform I bring home to dinner or visit in the hospital haven't, I find, ever been far from home before. They look around with curiosity; they hope to 'see the sights,' Broadway or Hollywood, for choice. But the way to bring a smile hovering around their lips, and a glint in their eyes, is to talk about the places that they do know. Missouri will laugh with you about its razorback hogs, its mules and persimmons. Alabama drawls a longing reference to red clay soil, to peachblow against blue spring sky, or cotton bolls when they begin to open; Utah talks of towns and green Mormon oases in a war-paint-colored desert. So you've never been to Arkansas? Mister, you ought to see something. You don't know North Dakota? And the eyes that look on it as home look at you with friendly pity.

In those eyes, at the back of each brain among the uniformed many, is some little scene that I shall never know. That glimpse of a fraction of the U.S.A. stands for the whole. It wouldn't make a striking picture postcard. But it's the one face, like the face a man keeps in his wallet. A lane through birch woods, its ruts familiar as beloved wrinkles? A hill pasture, with a roof of an old barn rising just over the grassy crown? A big tulip poplar and a house little beneath it, with a cow path through the summer grasses to the girl's house? I see all those places through the window of the train before the dark falls, but I'll never see them again. I'll forget them. Not so the boys who came from there, no matter where they go. And it may be a long, long way.

So, Baldur, let's put away the chessmen and fold up the board, and come out to the edge of the hill where this house stands. Here is the face of the land I daily live with. The very calls of the birds, mocker and western meadowlark and wren-tit, are now the sounds of home, and so are those church bells whose old clangor reaches us so mildly. I can tell you what time it is by the far-off rumble of the trains — the long orange-yellow trains that come thundering into town and out of it. I know the *Daylight* going up to San Francisco and the *Daylight* coming down and, awake in my bed, I can say, by its whistle, 'That's the *Lark*,' or 'That's the *Coaster*.' I can hear taps and reveille blown, faint but smart, down at the military hospital. There are its roofs, right over there toward the Marine flying-base, looking neat and new and uniform.

The rest of the town looks cheerfully casual by comparison. You see the roofs, from my doorstep, rising out of the trees. Those are my friends' houses, where the smoke, this brisk autumn morning, is curling up quietly. That's the house of Tom and Dorothy Ripley, who are always at home to friends for tea; there's my doctor's house; I went to college with him in the East and knew him only by sight then; he knows a great deal about my throat now, and his son and mine are rival patrol leaders in Mounted Troop 21, Mission Council, Santa Barbara, Boy Scouts of America. I always know when Jack's coming up to see Malcolm, because I hear the slow ring of his Palomino's hoofs on the mile-long lane winding up from their house to ours. Living here on a hill a thousand feet above the sea is like life in a medieval castle, in that you survey the demesne below like a lord, and when a knight comes riding you have time to think about him, before he arrives and hitches out by the old barn.

Those are the flying Marines now, coming over in formation, filling the hollow dome of the sky, long before you can see them, with their rumor; then it's a threat, then a roaring actuality, glittering in the sunlight overhead — and my boys dash out of the house, if they're home, to look up with worshiping faces and to argue vehemently the exact make of the planes. Now they are passing, past, a flight of hornets that seem in perspective to close in until they are one sting, vanishing, unseen, only a purposeful hum.

When your eyes come down from the sky they take in the mountains first, the rugged coast ranges, young and hard and pressing down close to the sea; they are clothed with an intricate scrub that we should have called *maquis* in the south of France, and here known as chaparral. But in the long canyons running seaward, like this at our feet, there are sycamores, and live-oaks — to a European, plane and ilex trees.

In such groves, you see, the town is built. It is cradled, almost fondled, in the brown palm of California, tipped a little to the froth of the sea.

There are many seas, says a California poet; there is only one great ocean. The Pacific is the greatest natural phenomenon upon the planet. The men who reached it here had come to the end of something, and there is nowhere now for America to go, beyond this point, except to the beginning of a new world.

America, as a nation of English-speaking people with a Protestant and a republican tradition, didn't get to Santa Barbara until 1847, but fifty years, to a day, after Columbus discovered America, one Rodriguez Cabrillo dropped anchor out there where the water is sparkling so blue between the kelp beds and the chain of those mountainous islands.

There is a striking difference between the arrival at the Bahamas of Columbus and the discovery of California by this Portuguese, Cabrillo. Columbus was looking for Asia; he bumped into America by accident, assumed for some time that he was in Japan, and died without ever having heard either the name America or the fact of the New World.

But Cabrillo came looking for California. He, and the Spaniards of his day, had read about an 'island' of this name, where there were pearls to be had for the picking up, and gold and beautiful maidens, and where the climate was delicious. It was all written down in *The Deeds of Esplandian*, a romance by a popular author named Ordoñez de Montalvo. Cervantes attributed the delusions of his poor friend Don Quixote to reading too much Montalvo. Where this high-colored romancer got the notion or the name of 'California' we do not know. His readers only asked how they could get there.

Cabrillo was the first to; an October day just four hundred years ago found his cockleshell rocking in those blue waters between us and the islands. Mysterious and inaccessible, that chain of submerged mountain peaks guards this coast and acts as a breakwater to protect the Santa Barbara Channel. Even before the Navy made them forbidden ground to the civilian, the islands were *terra incognita* to most of us. Few of my townsmen have ever set foot on those shores that gleam at us not forty miles away; I hungered to, when first I came to live here, but I've grown to enjoy the hunger more, perhaps, than I should the islands. For they are inhospitably craggy, fringed with reefs, and comparatively barren. The little Anacapa group is now a government sanctuary for nesting sea birds, and even in peacetime cannot be approached without special permission. Big Santa Cruz and its slightly smaller neighbor, Santa Rosa, are owned by a few ranchers; to land is to trespass. But those who have been allowed to go there speak of the sea caves, the deep glens filled with evergreen forests, the wildflowers and congregations of sea birds. San Miguel Island is accessible enough, since there is a colony of fishermen on it; but, sandy and swept by gales or wrapped in fog, it has allured few visitors, and whatever Coast Guard men may be posted out there must be lonely boys longing for liberty.

Cabrillo in his day found the islands populous with Canalino Indians. Each island had its own language and costumes and customs. All vied in the skill of their expert sailors and fishers and swimmers. No such big and seaworthy canoes as theirs were found elsewhere south of Oregon. For Cabrillo the islands held a fascination that ultimately proved fatal. While exploring, he fell from a cliff on Santa Rosa and broke his arm below the shoulder; either it was poorly set or he did not wait for it to heal before undertaking an arduous and ill-starred journey to the north; at any rate, he died on January 3, 1543, and was buried there on San Miguel. The sands have long since swallowed his forgotten grave. And, just a year or two ago, out at the county hospital that lies hidden by those northward hills, there died the last surviving member of the Channel Island tribes, at a great old age.

That drowsy clamor floating up a few minutes past came

from the bells of the Mission. Step out here along the canyon's rim and you can see it — there, those two low towers with rosy domes just rising above the sea of treetops. Out here in California we're proud of our missions, as you are of your minsters and castles. You see, six years and a day before the Liberty Bell pealed out the news of independence over the streets of young Philadelphia, another bell spoke, the breadth of the continent away. It spoke to wilderness, with a small lonely clapper. It said that Christ was even here, here on this arid and heathen shore. It called to the painted Indians who listened in hiding, to come. The man in the somber robe, pulling on the rope where the bell hung from a live-oak tree, was Father Junípero Serra, and he was founding the mission at Monterey.

That's the little seaport town where the American colors were run up to claim California from the Spanish. But long before, Father Serra had claimed it for God. Along *El Camino Real*, the King's Highway, were established twenty-one missions, a day's journey of forty miles apart — 'Father Serra's Rosary,' the pious called it. Ours we call the Queen of the Missions, for its beauty. The Brothers of Saint Francis founded it in 1786. When all the other Spanish missions of California had been secularized by the hostile civil government of Mexico, and the priests had fled, the good monks of Santa Barbara never quite gave up. Without funds, without help from the Church, there were, at the worst, at least two or three who clung on here through many decades, trying to save the buildings from ruin, guarding the old documents.

When the Americans came, the Franciscan brothers were welcomed back to their lovely place of worship. For long ago, before ever this republic was born, we had decided to bury religious quarrels; the embers may still smoulder a little, but we don't allow fools to blow on them. And I'd like to slip it in here that when the old law that disfranchised the Roman Catholics of England was at last repealed over there in the early nineteenth century, Protestant hands set our own Liberty Bell to ringing.

To most of us, the Mission down there doesn't belong so much to Rome as it does to the city of Santa Barbara. It is *our* Mission, the town's, and I should like to drive you very slowly past it, so that you could see the classic façade and the ruddy bloom of those two old domes against the looming blue of the coastal range.

One hot June morning a few years ago, when the monks were at their six o'clock Mass, the earth began to growl and the Mission floor to move under them. The altar decorations were flung into the chancel, but the priest exhorted the brothers to remain at prayer, and God must have guided him, for had they rushed out of the door they would have been caught by the fall of the adobe towers. While the monastery rooms were falling, the Father Superior dashed in and carried out on his shoulders the aged historian of the California missions, the invalid Father Zephyrin Engelhardt. But somehow the altar light (which, uniquely among all the missions', has never been extinguished since the founding) was still burning, and the old bells you hear are those that survived the shock.

The town was damaged too, but one of the first tasks of the whole community was to restore their mission. Protestants and Catholics alike gave money for this. One of the most zealous in raising it, they tell me, was a fellow who goes by the nickname of 'Heck,' a man I know who's got a successful insurance and real estate business just off State Street.

You'll meet him in a few minutes, Baldur, because I'm going to take you along now to a Rotary luncheon, at which I'll be only a guest myself. So put your monocle in your pocket, and open your mind even a little wider. It would do Heck a lot of good to know you, and you'll have to get to understand Heck if this country of ours is going to make sense to you.

Heck was born in the Middle West, like me and a great many other Californians, and had a public-school education and a year in a state university before he was called in the draft of 1917, got pneumonia in training camp, was sent overseas, just missed by a torpedo off Nantes, and billeted in a French village that had twice been occupied by the Germans and was pretty well shattered as to roofs, nerves, and population. After thinking he would never get a crack at those Heinies, and growing mad enough at the French to have fought them instead, Heck was rushed into a forest patch in the Argonne, where his behavior earned fully as much respect as I have for your intellect, Baldur. Though nobody gets to see his decoration except his wife and three children.

When he got home, I understand, he didn't feel like going back to State U. He wasn't a college boy any more; on the other hand, the war had snatched from him whatever special training he might have got through education, and the long perspective offered by the humanities. He was dumped into the great pool of the unemployed and swam bravely out of it. He had left to him, intact, all his personal ideals, but he had lost all the impersonal idealism he went to war with. Having gone overseas with a vague idea that he was righting the wrongs done Jeanne d'Arc, or at least redeeming a debt to Lafayette, he heard now that many Frenchmen and many Germans believed he had gone over to redeem the investments of the House of Morgan. And though he didn't think so himself, he'd been sold somehow; he grew more and more sure of it. President Wilson's name to him became a sorry laugh. The League of Nations was a trick we'd seen through. America's coastline was an invincible wall around the best damn country in the world.

Heck came to California in accordance with a tradition now three hundred years old that an American goes west. For there are three great movements in American history. There's the westward push which began the minute the first settlers landed and is now carrying men, flag, and ideals across the Pacific. There is the American Revolution, which began in the democratic struggles of Americans' ancestors a thousand years ago, and is now rising to a crisis. And there is the spectacle that astounds and confounds the world, of the welding together — into one nation, one people — the descendants of Europeans, Asiatics, Africans, and redskins.

Heck is daily involved in these titanic movements. They bewilder him as much as they do you and me. To cope with them, he seeks earnestly to find out what he believes is good and what is dangerous or sheer poppycock. Many of his beliefs are inherited prejudices, but no easily followed line separates these from the faiths of his fathers which have guided us this far.

Heck was waiting for me at the door of the room where the Rotarians were going to have their luncheon. Doctors, bakers, real estate and insurance men, my tailor, my dentist, my lawyer, were all streaming in. To you, Baldur, who understand café leisure, it would appear that they were hurrying, but they were taking an unusual amount of time for lunch. They might be in this room an hour and a half, which was three times as much as most would ordinarily give themselves at noon. They had not come, exactly, to hear me, but for twenty minutes they were going to listen to me. I found this more flattering than I would the attention of an audience which might be paying me to divert them for a full hour. These men, on the terms of equals, for some reason wanted to know what I thought.

This might have impressed me with myself but for the easy turning of the wheels of Rotary. Its friendliness is determined. Fraternalism is sacrosanct; they fine a member, you know, if he doesn't use a given or nick-name. There is no trouble in knowing a fellow's intimate monicker, because it is writ large on a lapel badge the size of a butter-plate. So my doctor turned into 'Hank' and my dentist into 'Jack' and my lawyer, who is a suave worldling, into 'Shorty.' This would be bewildering at best to a person of reserved manners and retired life; it horrifies and amuses my friends of the sort who skip out of church by a side door so that the beauty of the service won't be ruined for them by having to shake hands with the minister. However, I got my training for it in a college fraternity made up, for the great good of my soul, largely of young men whom I would never have picked for bosom brothers if I had not been flung in their arms by the fraternal order. A little out of practice now, I struck out for the opposite shore and, if my form was poor, the water was fine.

When at our speakers' table Heck got up to introduce me to townsmen who already knew me in one way or another, I could tell from his face that he was worried. I'd given him my subject, 'Let's Get On with the American Revolution.' Now the revolutions that we have seen in the last twenty years look like everything we hope is un-American. The horrors of the excesses of the Bolshevist upheaval in Russia shocked us all, and that assault on religion and private property disgusted Heck not only because men must live by religion and property, but because the State in Russia had become master over man. Americans have never had in their heads or hearts the image of the State with a capital S. The Germans have never been without such a concept before their eyes, so that when the Nazi revolution came along Heck saw, as clearly as Thomas Jefferson would have seen, that no benefits that an all-powerful State can confer upon an all-subservient individual are worth the single thing it took away from him.

And of course Heck had been taught in school to believe that the American Revolution began when the embattled farmers fired the shot heard round the world, and that it ended at Yorktown. He finds it easy and safe to approve of our Revolution in the past, to put up monuments to long-dead heroes and historic battles. It was safe and easy, too, I said, to be a Tory in the year of Valley Forge. I said that the War of Independence was only an early battle, and that our Revolution of Democracy has no more than fairly got under way; here in the United States it is in its first great glory, a springtime more than one hundred and fifty years long. I said that the Atlantic Charter was really a Declaration of Interdependence, and that as a nation we'd already signed it. Our lives, our fortunes, and our sacred honor are pledged as thoroughly as theirs were by John Hancock and Button Gwinnett.

Now Heck would give his life for anything big enough; he's a braver man than I am. When he sees somebody in want, he gives his money; he is the biggest giver in the history of the world. His word is as good as that of anybody you can name, just because he is so reluctant about giving it. And that badge on his lapel denies that he is provincial, in however small a town you may find him, because Rotary has internationalism written into its creed, just as race prejudice is written out.

But it's no fun, when you've survived one world war and reached an easy middle age, to be told yours is the bold and dangerous rôle of the revolutionary patriot. Because a revolution hits everybody in the country where he lives. It isn't fought solely or even principally on a battle front, but right in your home, in your mind and your heart. You have to leave the side that seemed safe and looked right, if you're going to become a revolutionary.

I told Heck, in front of everybody, that I was scareder of the revolution than he is, because I'm not so brave. The cause of our great Democratic Revolution will not honor me, I presume, by asking for my life; I'm too old and soft. It may ask, though, for the precious lives of my sons; it may claim my peace of mind and pleasant living; it may ask me to love those I have never understood, enough to treat them as brothers. It may be that before we can, in the words of the framers of the Constitution, insure domestic tranquillity, provide for the common defense, promote the general welfare, and secure the blessings of liberty, we shall have to lift others from the ground where they have been beaten by their brutal overseers.

Worse, it may be that another dreadful conflict is to be sustained. For the great wheels of history are rolling faster and farther, whether we like it or not. That's what revolution is, a turning over, the kind of turning that gets you forward.

And unless we leap to direct this revolution that started 'way back, perhaps with Magna Carta, the wheels which have gathered such terrible momentum may crash over us and crush us.

9

The Trail to Transylvania

THE MAN AND THE TREE stood each in the other's path. The man, staring up at the tree, hefted the axe in his grip consideringly. The tree was a tulip poplar, the tallest he had ever seen, and he had seen some trees in his time. Now in the early spring morning it cast a long shadow across his way. He had paced that shadow, and measured his own; the rule of three was the farthest boundary of his mathematical knowledge, and he worked it now. Since his shadow was to his stature as the tree's shadow was to its giant height, he calculated that this tulip poplar towered nigh on two hundred feet.

At the level of his eyes the bark was deeply furrowed with age. Tipping back his head, his far-seeing gaze traveled up the bole, that for half its height rose straight as a flagpole, unbranching. Where the branches gushed out, the tree was younger; they made a mighty frame for summer's canopy, bare now in the March light except for the bleached bracts where last year's cones had fallen out. Those upright cups looked like gutted candlesticks waiting to be filled and lighted again, with blossoms like pale red and yellow water lilies. Straight up and up soared the leader stem, the bark of it growing satiny and nearly white, too slim for bearing, free and high and happy-looking, like a man's daughter before she comes to wed.

The Trail to Transylvania

The man swept the downward length of the tree with a quick glance and whistled his admiration softly. Then a twig broke in the forest behind him, and even his skin seemed to listen. After a minute of aboriginal silence the hoofbeats sounded so that even another man than this could have heard them. Then a rider came in sight; his horse was lathered and showed green foam on the bit.

'We're to go,' he shouted, as he pulled up. 'The Colonel says blaze away at the trail, Dan'l.'

The man with the axe rubbed a knuckle on his chin, and sheltered the spark in his eyes with his lids as if from the wind rising in him.

'Is the treaty signed yet with the Cherokees?'

'Won't be for a week, I'd say, the way old Dragging Canoe is speechifying. But it's a sure thing. So the Colonel says, go.'

What the Colonel said went. Richard Henderson, a self-made man, an able lawyer and ex-judge, was accustomed to relying on his own judgments and initiatives; he had what promoters call vision. And what he had seen was the dream he called Transylvania, a fortune beyond the forest, the biggest land deal in history.

In those days just before the Revolution, many were hungering for that unexplored Canaan known to the Indians as Caintuck, 'Among-the-meadows.' But King George had forbidden his American subjects to set foot there. Those choice lands he was holding perhaps to distribute to favorites at court, or at royal prices to London land syndicates. To Americans themselves, Kentucky was forbidden ground. Yet a few had been there, on pain of the law and at risk of their lives, covering their traces, smothering their campfires, hiding their trap lines, fearing sometimes to fire a shot in those primeval depths.

In Henderson's early forties he fell in to talk with one of these few, a mild-mannered man by the name of Boone. This Dan Boone had a farm over on the Yadkin that wasn't yielding much, a pack of handsome but hungry children, a trump of a wife named Rebecca, a long rifle-gun that he called Tick-Licker, a longer debt sheet for powder, shot, and traps, and a string of the tallest tales ever told. Tales you wanted to believe, of a land beyond the dark forest, where the meadows were like velvet and the black loam went down to China. Tales of ten-tined elk and richest beaver fur, that you had to believe because Boone had the hides and antlers to show you. Boone had eyes, too, that seemed to see a long way. He didn't have much of a head for business, and it's true that his life long he never got the hang of land claims and always lost out in the end. But he had seen what was to become Kentucky; he had seen the way the nation must grow, and deep in his simple heart he believed himself divinely appointed to guide the settlers forth.

The Colonel hired him. It wasn't hard for a popular promoter like Henderson to find eight other investors to capitalize 'Henderson's Transylvania Company.' Nor was it hard to find two score or more of men to follow anywhere that Dan Boone led. Young men, strong with an axe, quick with a trigger, landless in the crowding settlements, jobless in their stifled commerce, too long for their beds, too tall for the old home roof. Henderson's advertisement brought them flocking.

It brought too, a sharp protest from the royal governors of North Carolina and Virginia. They denounced the new Company on solid grounds of British law. Lawyer Henderson knew the ins and outs of that. But he saw there was a revolution coming, and British law might be thrown out. When the storm troubled the waters, he might land his enormous fish.

So off he went, to bargain with the Tennessee Cherokees. A thousand redskins came to view the red paint, beads, none-so-pretties, firewater, tomahawks, and other bait offered. Against their value, the grave chiefs pondered the worth of the northern hunting grounds — twenty million acres, or about half of all Kentucky, lying between the Ohio and the Cumberland, the Cumberland Mountains and the Kentucky River. After days of powwow under the sycamores, the Treaty of Watauga was signed, and red men and white feasted in celebration.

Dan Boone was ready and waiting, twenty-six miles away at the Long Island in the Holston River. With him were thirty picked axemen. When the order came from Henderson, on March 10, 1775, Dan spat on his palms, grasped his axe, swung it glinting in spring sunshine over his head, and struck the first blow on the Wilderness Trail.

Behind him other axes rang. There was a laugh on the lips of the woodsmen from deep in their chests. The brooks and the birds, uncorked by spring, sang together. Ahead lay a boundless future and if there was danger in it, why so were there powder and lead. Over Bay Mountain the trail-breakers cut their way, and down the valley of the Clinch and across it. The chiming clang of their blades mocked a silence older than Adam. The sons of Adam were here now, sending down in a toppling fall the walls against them that had been centuries growing. Over Clinch Mountain they cleared a path, down into the valley of the Powell and a long way beside its rugged course. It rushed laughing beside them and ahead of them, and beckoned with the glint of its next curve shining through the forest. Down crashed the rooted giants in the way these men chose to take. Up Powell's Mountain they hacked and they hewed, and through the Cumberland Gap, where they stopped, leaning on their axe helves, and then with a laugh at the ache in their backs started down on the other side, their heels on Kentucky soil at last. They had come more than one hundred miles in less than a week!

Here utter wilderness began. In the intricate glens, over razorback ridges, a way must be found, cut clean of tangling vines so ancient that their stems were thick as a leg; logs must be lifted from the way, boggy spots filled, streams bridged by timbers felled and placed; every mile a tree was blazed. Beyond the gorge of the Rockcastle, Boone encountered twenty miles of dead brush, time-hardened, and timbers fallen in jackstraw chaos. He always swore this was the worst; he had to burn his way through this Sleeping Beauty tangle with torches; then he and his men passed like a crackling wind through the giant canebrake. By night Indians attacked, slaying some of the trail-makers as they slept. Faint-of-hearts fled back. But only two weeks from the time they left the Long Island, the dauntless survivors stood, with quivering muscles and sweat-blinded eyes, gazing in triumph on what one of the party calls 'the pleasing and rapturous plains of Kentucky,' the future Bluegrass region where 'a new sky and a strange earth seemed presented to the view.'

Slim as a cowpath, dangerous as a tightrope, the Wilderness Trail was the path to America's future. A rich man could ride it horseback; a poor man must walk it, pulling or packing his goods. Many a poor woman trod it, many a barefoot child. Probably two hundred thousand American feet had tramped it before the day Henry Clay stopped upon it and appeared to listen. Asked what for, he said, 'For the millions yet to come.'

The American people, De Tocqueville observes, do not see the mighty wilderness they are destroying; they give no thought to the trees they fell or the deer they slay; what they see is the crops they will grow there, the cattle they will raise there, and the rooftrees that will rise there over the heads of their children. He considered us the most practical people in the world and, in the old European sense, the least poetic. But, himself a man of breadth and vision, he saw that there was a new kind of poetry born out of our soil — the poetry of the future. It would not come only from the lips of recognized poets; the Muse herself was to be democratized so that there would be a little bit of this poetry in everyone.

Boone had his fragment. He could barely spell; he read sign better than print, and he called the prairie the 'purarie,' in writing and doubtless in speech. But, faithful to De Tocqueville's picture of the woodsman, he believed that God had appointed him to drive away the cruel, treacherous, filthy, and ignorant savage from His fairest province, that the smoke of good men's chimneys might rise safely in the clearings.

It's true that he didn't practice forest conservation; would you, with an Indian behind every tree? He shot does as well as bucks, and he hunted and trapped in all seasons. It wasn't until he got his wish — to hear Kentucky-born babies laughing and cocks crowing where the Shawnees had whooped — that a great sadness came over him, and he realized that he understood more about the vanishing bears than the advancing land-lawyers. So wearily he sought wilderness again, on the 'puraries' of Missouri, and there in his long old age watched the young men pass his door, going west on the Santa Fé and Oregon Trails.

I've gone west too, you'll remember, putting my dauntless wife into my covered Buick, and I took care to go the way Boone went. The Wilderness Road originally ran up the Shenandoah, though this was not the part that Boone cut; this portion was completed before his day. But the Shenandoah Valley is all part of the same epic, the westward rolling of the American stream. This epic, greater than Homer's or Virgil's, is known to all of us; we feel it in our bones, and when we say a name like 'Shenandoah,' or 'the Natchez Trace,' or 'the Comanche Trail,' or 'the Columbia,' we groove a little deeper the channel that our national legend takes. The legends of America differ from those of Europe because we have no need to borrow from the supernatural; tall men are enough to make our tall tales good. Lincoln is a legend, Boone is a legend, and so are Stonewall Jackson, Walt Whitman, Kit Carson, Mark Twain. I call them so because when we run out of the voluminous facts about them, we lovingly supply what is true enough in spirit at least.

So the Shenandoah is a legend, one of beauty. Those gentlemen adventurers, the Knights of the Golden Horseshoe, riding over the Blue Ridge in 1716, were among the first who gazed upon that valley in its virgin fertility. John Bartram, Quaker and botanist to George III, was the earliest to stand waist-high among its unplucked flowers. He called it 'my valley,' and would not tell others how to reach it. But you cannot keep a secret like the Shenandoah.

Today the Shenandoah means apple blossoms and apples, peach-blow and peaches, plum-bloom and plum and pears. These flowering trees were puffs of light when I came rolling by; the rusty red floor of the valley — green where the fields were springing — lay wide and fertile between the long marching ranges. Meadowlark song rang all down this corridor forty miles wide and three hundred miles long. It seems the happiest of places, but not if you remember. For the true legends of the Shenandoah are filled with old echoes of war, of the armies of Stonewall Jackson and Phil Sheridan marching and countermarching and clashing here; here the boys of a military school came out of their classrooms to hold a desperate line; here Sheridan swore so to ravage the resources and communications of the valley that a crow would have to carry its rations. And here Robert E. Lee, after surrendering the Confederate armies and refusing every sort of lucrative and honorary post, accepted the presidency of a war-shattered college with only forty pupils in it, and thereby showed the South how proudly the humbled might begin to build again.

When you get to the headwaters of the Shenandoah, you turn west, if like me you're following the Wilderness Road, and you go up over the ridges of the Alleghenies; the legend of Boone haunts every mile, and the Boone men are still coming out of the mountains to whup whoever needs it. We picked one up in the extreme southwest or lower left-hand corner of the gable which is the homelike shape of Virginia. He was a Kentuckian, a soldier, and if I wanted to know how the men at Boone's back looked and talked and thought, I had only to meet this fellow.

It took all my attention to understand his English (the reiterated word 'thole' I presently understood to mean what I pronounce as 'told'). He hardly bothered to understand my English, as I was a foreigner who would soon be rolling out of these mountains. But before I went he was going to offer me the hospitality of the finest yarns he knew. They were all about fights; he began point-first with the blow or the murder, and unraveled backward the aimless explanation of how it all started. He came from Harlan County, and I opined mildly that they raised 'em tough there. He protested. 'They kill a lot more men in the next county to ourn.' Fourteen when he went to work in the coal mines, he was seventeen when he enlisted, and twenty now. His eyes, which had seen so much and so little, made me flinch; they had a kind of innocent deadliness in them, the look of a man who could kill highheartedly, out of pure, disinterested love of it. The German or the Jap that meets him is as out of luck as a Shawnee.

He left us beyond the Rockcastle, which has earned its name by carving into crenelated keeps the sweetening soft limestones of Kentucky. Here where his ancestors had helped Boone blaze a way through the worst of the wilderness, the private set jauntily off afoot to see his family, before crossing the ocean that he had never yet beheld. And we rolled comfortably on, past the spot where Kit Carson was born, to the end of Dan Boone's road and into the heart of the Bluegrass.

The Bluegrass country is an open, rolling plateau, just north and east of the center of Kentucky. The rivers have plowed easily through its limestones, and so lie between beautiful cliffs. It's in dispute whether the grass that the English call spear grass was also aboriginally native here, or later introduced, but Boone saw great herds of buffalo, and so there was some sort of grass here from the beginning. Now it appears to be all pasture. The bluegrass clothes this earth from the edge of the road to the sills of the doors, and horses crop it right up to the threshold of the finest mansion. A horse in the Bluegrass, a good horse, is accorded the honors of the noblest of guests and allowed the privileges of the bestloved of children. The sheen of love is on the very hides of these horses, and they lift their heads like lords happy to be your servant.

The good stock of Kentucky is not all horseflesh. As fast as the bluegrass grows, it is turned into cream by Guernsey and Jersey. They look as content as the long-haired black Angus cattle look wild and improbable in that lush placidity. The sheep are Cheviot and Southdown; now in April the fat lambs, in sudden capering access of appetite, butted at the nipples of their mothers, fell to their knees to suckle, under the curve of maternal bulk, and wriggled their woolly tails in first and simplest ecstasy. The hogs had young too, looking, in the brief charm of their infancy, almost dainty in that setting of velvet green. The cocks were proud of their breed; the turkey gobbler spread his fantastic male display of beauty like a Sultan.

For years I have been discoursing about the rightness and the greatness of American wilderness. I belong to a Wilderness Society dedicated to the preservation of aboriginal conditions. I send telegrams to congressmen to save the redwoods and save the antelope and save the ivory-billed woodpecker — which requires many square miles of uninhabited swamp timber to support it — and I have traveled to the farthest limits of my country looking for places that man has not defiled. But man in the Bluegrass adorns the Nature of which he has possessed himself. A kinder sky, a sweeter earth, a friendlier people, a fatter yield, a seemlier outlook there are not in this world. Dan Boone's fondest dreams have more than come true. He was right, and if there had been a Wilderness Society then to oppose him, it would have been wrong.

For sleep we turned aside to Shakertown, or what is left of it. This deserted village is hard by Harrodsburg, but they are no more alike than a gray little spinster aunt is like a lively family. James Harrod came over the Kentucky mountains in the same year as Boone; his town stood somewhat in rivalry to Boonesborough. Boone's town is gone, but you can today, if you wish, go over to Harrodsburg in season for the races. For your true Bluegrass town has got its racetrack, as Spanish towns have bullrings and Italian towns have opera houses. And Harrodsburg had the first track in the state of Kentucky. Racing is the local sport and industry, and belongs to the local people. But Shakertown on its hill was built to last forever by a people who would take no chances even on posterity. They practiced complete celibacy, and in consequence of the success which the old folks achieved, and of the notable apostasy of the younger members, there is now not a Shaker left in Shakertown.

So much the better for us, we thought. For one of their cluster of austere empty dwellings among the meadows had been made into a place of public entertainment. My wife, who likes best an inn with everybody out, found it just what she likes and was vastly entertained by the two front doors, one for the Shaker men and one for the Shaker women, and by the double stairs that chastely mount on opposite sides of the handsome plain hall, to the floor where the airy chambers are.

So, late in the still April evening, we solemnly took our separate ways up the broad old treads — and met at the top. I thought, as I lay in my bed that night, I could smell the violets I had seen in the Shaker yard below. I knew I was on the scent of something old yet young, something full of April. Tomorrow, I promised myself, I would look for the vanished capital of a state that never was — the site of Boonesborough, in Transylvania. And there, I hoped, I would find some footprint of the girl who had gone ahead of me all this day, Dan Boone's daughter, Jemima.

With her mother Rebecca, she was the first bit of white womanhood ever to take the Wilderness Trail. For Dan Boone came back, that first Kentucky summer of 1775, to fetch his family from beyond the mountains; you hadn't tamed wilderness, to his mind, till you planted your women in it. He had to wait for Rebecca to have the next baby, and then he had to delay to build it a coffin. After that they started. Jemima was thirteen at the time; she and her little brother, Daniel Morgan Boone, kicked heels in the flanks of their horses to see who would be first on the trail their daddy had cleared, first to ride out on the soil of Kentucky. It was late August; the leaves would have been full then, hanging still in the breathless heat, hiding redbird and black bear and Shawnee. Tradition says that, her dolls outgrown, Jemima carried a panther kitten with her. Facts proved she was a panther kitten herself. She was such a little beauty, even then, that men turned to stare at her. I, for my part, had long been looking over my shoulder at Dan Boone's fearless daughter before — a hundred and sixty-seven years too late — I came seeking Boonesborough.

10

Dan Boone's Daughter

SIX FEET FOUR, WITH legs and arms like limbs of ironwood, cradling his rifle, a long knife in his belt and a long look in his jet-black eyes, James Harrod strode through the sycamores and fresh-leaving elms. He was coming to Boonesborough, and he knew by the lowing of cattle in the woods, the calling of crows and the storming of pigeon flocks, by the rifle shots and the smell of woodsmoke, that he was getting near Henderson's town. It certainly wasn't much like Daniel Boone to be advertising his presence like this, shooting up all the game in the country, and never a sentinel posted. Why, Harrod might have been old Blackfish himself, or Big Jim who had tortured to death Dan's son James on Wallen Ridge, for all the settlers in Boonesborough heeded his coming. Dan'l knew better than this. What were they thinking of? Land, he guessed, and money come easy and quick, Colonel Henderson's way. And when a man thinks he's going to be rich as a king tomorrow, he acts like riches was the same as salvation — you can plumb forget all your good sense for the little time you've got to linger in this vale of tears.

The long stride crossed trout-lily patches and low purple larkspur, with never a sound. Over at Harrodsburg men had land too, enough for their needs. Maybe they hadn't bought their claims from the Cherokees with a fancy treaty;

they hadn't bought 'em from the bears either, or the wildcats;
they'd just staked 'em and worked 'em. They'd raised their
cabin walls and cleared their patches and planted their corn.
And now this lawyer Henderson and his outfit of 'Proprietors'
claimed to own that very land, or leastways every foot around
the settlements. So now the grim shadow of tall James Harrod,
stepping into the clearing, fell on the wild grass around
Boonesborough.

Why, the place warn't even stockaded yet! And they here
a month past! But Henderson and his speculators had got
the whole shebang staked out into lots, he saw. Their cabins
not half finished, either, and they a-getting rich on paper
buying and selling to each other and buying back again!
So the tale of it had come to Harrodsburg. Well, it was a fine
place for a town, here in a holler at the bend o' the Kentucky,
and he wished Boone well; over at Harrodsburg they were
mighty obleeged to him for his Trail and glad he was in the
neighborhood. Harrodsburg and Boonesborough, Floyd's
outfit over to St. Asaph's, Logan at Logan's Station, they'd all
swap powder and vittles, and they'd come to each other's aid
any time it was needful. But the land grab of this here
Transylvania Company — that was something different from
a staked claim that a man worked hard to earn. It didn't
seem right to James Harrod to bite off more'n you could
chew, maybe, or needed to fill your belly.

He gave three loud halloos, for it's bad manners and poor
strategy, in any wilderness, to walk in unannounced. Dan
Boone, a few days later, happened to mention this in a letter;
it's dated May 19, 1775, and when in the fort at Harrodsburg
I puzzled out the blotted and faded ink I found myself winc-
ing a little, as if at a Shawnee arrow past my ear. 'Dear Sir,'
wrote Dan to one Charles Telfridge, Esquire,

> The Powder and Ball I received and it come to hand when
> needed. I could not reach you before you left, but I am pleased
> with the work we have done here. I feel sure we can hold
> against a huge number of savages. In coming in, signal as be-

fore. I hope to be living when you arrive, to see you. I found signs of savages this day. I shall say nothing. I am, Dear Sir, Yours, Daniel Boone.

Colonel Richard Henderson, donning his coat of red velvet with gold lacing, met the accusing James Harrod adroitly. The claims of all settlers, Harrodsburg's included, would in point of law be worthless, he smoothly brought out, if Caintuck remained a westernmost extension of Virginia. For legally, he smilingly admitted, nobody could make a treaty with the Indians, nobody could buy from them, except King George's governors. But, he suggested, offering snuff out of a gold box, all claims could be made good if the settlers themselves set up a new government and got it recognized by the Continental Congress. The scheme for that, he assured James Harrod, was ready, prepared by the Proprietors of the Transylvania Company.

The proposed state of Transylvania was the boldest attempt at monopolistic government ever made upon American soil. Having snapped up half of Kentucky at a quarter of a cent an acre, the Company offered it at around thirteen and a half cents an acre, plus quit-rents of fifty cents an acre yearly. Quit-rent being something the purchaser is never quit of, the Proprietors were thereby assured of rich annuities. Before 1775 was over, five hundred and sixty thousand acres had been sold. Some lands, great blocks of the best, were never opened to sale; the Proprietors quietly reserved these to themselves. And still there remained about nineteen million acres offered on the market.

Disposition of lots at Boonesborough was made by drawing for them; since nobody is ever satisfied with what he gets by lot, the drawings, the scramble, the speculations, went heedlessly on. Dan Boone shook his head, for he knew the wilderness. Not by drawing lots was it to be won, not by speculation. Weeks it was taking these land-greedy men to get the simplest stockade completed, nor were the blockhouses all up. As for a well — What's the matter with the river, Dan? they asked him. Or rain barrels? And they went back to their land deals and dickerings.

So Dan was glad to see Jim Harrod; that must have been a handclasp! For these were men as hard in sinew as they were milk-mild, babe-innocent under the guidance of the deft and learned Judge Henderson. He acted quickly and, I suppose, all in good faith according to his own way of thinking. He called the first session of the 'House of Delegates of Transylvania,' to frame the constitution of this dreamed-up state, upon May 23, 1775. Men from the other settlements too arrived as delegates, earnest about business they did not quite understand. For council-hall, for capitol dome, they had a mighty elm; it was four feet through at the trunk, which at nine feet from the ground gave forth its vaulting branches. The floor for their debate was a carpet of white clover that rippled to the roots of the tree. Here innocence, serenity, a reverence-breeding antiquity, cast their influence on the proceedings. Setting down rifles and jugs, doffing coonskin caps, these forest heroes opened with prayer the first independent legislature to operate west of the mountains.

The simple delegates thereafter enacted rule-of-thumb laws to meet their frontier needs. Some laws provided courts, some decreed punishments for criminals. A militia was to be raised for mutual help. Fading records show that Boone brought in bills to conserve the game, and to improve the range and breed of horses. But when they came to a basic plan of government for Transylvania, the woodsmen were out of their depth. Respectfully they turned to listen to Judge Henderson.

The Colonel was ready; smoothly his scheme of government was run through, weighted heavily with advantage to the Proprietors. Three legislative houses were set up: the delegates of the people; a council of landowners, never to exceed twelve; and the Proprietors themselves. The second and third of these lawmaking bodies overlapped or had similar interests, so that it followed that about a dozen men, most of whom had 'bought in' to office for life, would control two thirds of the power of Transylvania, let the people increase as they might. Nor had the people apparently any chance to vote on the resolutions of the Proprietors. How this would have worked out was proved four months later when, safely back on the seaboard, the Proprietors were to resolve that anyone finding gold, silver, lead, iron, or sulphur on Transylvanian lands must yield half-interest in it to the Proprietors; that the Proprietors appoint one of their number to represent Transylvania by a seat in Congress; and that the price of Transylvanian land be sharply increased on January 1, 1776. In short, though the common people — as Transylvania's constitution called them — hadn't seen it yet, this was government of the people by the stockholders for the stockholders. The true color of it was given away by Henderson's revival of a picturesque feudal rite: the transfer of a bit of that clover-sweet turf from the hand of the Cherokees' lawyer to the Judge's own represented, to the awed woodsmen, the transfer of the demesne of Kentucky, all according to the ancient ceremony of 'Livery of Seisin.'

But in the colonies a storm was rising and, aware of it, the Proprietors prepared for safety, whichever way the wind might blow. In their constitution they protested Transylvania's sympathy with the Revolution, but they also slipped in an avowal of loyalty to King George — just in case. The Continental Congress had more decided views; no seat, it proved, was to be found for any delegate from this would-be state of Transylvania.

The political and financial outlook for Transylvania was thus so gloomy that Henderson hastened to Williamsburg, then the capital of Virginia, to lobby for his project. One by one the other Proprietors returned from Boonesborough until none was left there; all seemed to have business somewhere else. Theirs was the vision, and they had blocked out the structure of the economy and politics of Transylvania. They left it to the 'common people' — their customers who had bought the land — to finish the little details of felling the forest, raising crops, holding off the Indians, and otherwise improving the property.

I have read a historian who says that Boone was a pawn put forward by the true settler of Kentucky, Colonel Richard Henderson. I can only say that it was from Boone that Henderson first heard of the possibilities of Caintuck. He employed Daniel to clear the way for him and the other investors; the payment was in land, based on the title in the treaty with the Indians, a title which lawyer Henderson knew to be illegal. Subsequently, the Transylvania Company was granted by the legislature of Virginia a handsome tract near the present town of Henderson, in recognition of their enterprise. But Daniel Boone was to leave Kentucky landless, his claims pre-empted by those canny enough to get them validated before leaving seaboard Virginia. Then the owners were to come over the Wilderness Trail and push Dan farther west.

I have seen at Boonesborough a monument which vaunts the enterprise, devotion, vision, and daring of the Proprietors, perpetuating their names forever in granite. Boone's is down among the common people. Kentucky, I heard, is burned up about this monument. But Boone seems in the best of company, to me.

Boonesborough, when I found it, was a patch of violets; it was a twist of sparrow song; it was a budding twig, and a rotting log. It was a hollow among hills; it was a memory held in the crooked arm of the Kentucky River. Even the graves of Boonesborough's dead have been erased from sight by the floods of many springtimes. And here was spring again, come back as it came in 1776 when Jemima Boone was fourteen years old.

It's a fine pleasant thing to be fourteen, and pretty and healthy, and to have a man of twenty wanting to marry you, Colonel Calloway's nephew Flanders, with a tract of wilderness land for his own. It must have been better still to have Dan Boone for a strong and doting father, and Rebecca, wise in woman ways, to bring you up. And it must have been best of all to set your bare heels in the sweet earth of Kentucky in the days that were as the first morning of the world.

Those bare heels were the cause of all the trouble. For Jemima, running like a child, brought one foot down on a sharp stake of cane stubble. The cut nagged and burned her for days; the July weather was hot, and now she proposed to cool her foot in the river. Her playmates, Betsy Calloway, aged sixteen, and Betsy's sister Fanny, two years younger, knew as well as Jemima that they had no business to take the canoe and go paddling down the river. But it was Sunday, and you know what a Sunday afternoon is in midsummer. Dan Boone was napping in the cabin with his moccasins off; Colonel Calloway was reading, and Flanders hadn't been allowed by Daniel to court Jemima yet, and so was not hanging around her. That was to prove unfortunate for Dan's peace of mind.

The girls were as quiet as mischief about getting away in the boat, Jemima trailing her Achilles' heel in this wilderness Styx. But the Styx does not like those who embark upon it to return. Slyly it carried the boat downstream, and then when it had the girls out of earshot of the fort, it drew them against the opposite bank shadowed by a cliff. Even today you can't look at that other shore without remembering the threat of that cliff, the great woods that once crowned it, and the thick cane — a native bamboo — that crowded down to the water's edge. For that land over there was Shawnee country. The writ of Transylvanian law ran no farther there than a bullet sped, and though there hadn't been much trouble with the Indians yet at Boonesborough, Fanny was a goose to suggest going ashore there for wildflowers.

Jemima shook her head, flinging her hair out of her hot neck, and said with a laugh, 'No, I'm afraid of the Yellow Boys.'

Remember that her elder brother had been tortured to death by the Shawnee Big Jim, and that her father had hidden her in a hollow sycamore so she wouldn't meet the same fate. She had seen skeletons on the Wilderness Trail, and heard her daddy tell how some of the finest troops from Europe were cut to pieces at Braddock's defeat in the wilderness, where Washington was wounded and he, Dan Boone, and Dan Morgan, who had been young wagoners to the Continentals, had cut the traces of their horses and fled with the rest. Jemima's father was not a man to laugh when he said he was afraid of the Indians.

Jemima had a little, at least, of his good sense. She tried, with the other girls, to get the canoe back against the current and over a sandbar. But bronze hands, reaching out from the canebrake, helped the river; a Shawnee ran out to drag the boat shoreward and received on his head a thwack so hard that little Fanny's paddle was broken off in her hand. Screams in the three young throats were choked there by the threat of lifted tomahawks, and soon the forested steep hills, with the leaves hanging still and heavy and the pewee calling, hid what had been done.

Every American small boy has played at Indians. Even in France I used to see schoolboys in their black aprons trotting to the tobacconist's with a *sou*, to buy another chapter of the perpetual saga of *les peaux rouges*. Hollywood pours out good and bad redskin-bit-the-dust pictures, to meet our insatiable hunger. It's a dead heart that doesn't skip a beat when the eagle-feathered chief, shading his eyes, catches sight of the wagon train in the valley below. But familiarity with this legend makes it difficult for us to filter out the pleasing thrills and get to the pure horror of Indian fighting. To approximate it, combine guerilla warfare, as practiced by the most vengeful of the conquered, with the brutality of the conquerors, add the most fanatic hatred between races, pile on the instinct of the wolf-pack, and remember that both Indians and whites were fighting for their homes and their lands, their women and babies.

Viewed from the Indians' side, this war — which began as

soon as white men came claiming the Indians' country and the rights of a master race — was a fight for survival against invasion. The American Indian may well complain that his hospitality was abused when it was extended, that the treaties he made with us were repeatedly broken, that he was cheated and corrupted and, as a people with its own culture, exterminated. True that he didn't fight like a gentleman; he took the logical view that our babies were baby rattlesnakes. He agreed with Dan Boone that a white woman would civilize the wilderness faster even than her frontier husband, and it was civilization he had to fear.

The hatchet is buried now, and looking back we see the Indian wars as fought between two kinds of fellow Americans. We're proud of our redskins for the scrap they put up, and we speak of them in the tones that a sailor uses when he talks of a gale, or a hunter when he tells you about the grizzly that clawed him.

And of course Boone didn't have to put himself in the way of Indian trouble. He could have stayed at home in North Carolina and plowed his thin red clays and raised weaker crops and weedy children. He could have hunted rats in the barn with Tick-Licker; he could have saved to pay his taxes, and acknowledged himself the true and loyal subject of His Majesty George III. He could have gone to the tavern tap for adventure, and to jail for his debts. The small world of colonial America was well equipped with pews, pillories, clerks of the court, and threats of hellfire.

But over the Blue Ridge and beyond the Great Smokies and through the Cumberland Gap lay freedom. A great wilderness of it, enough liberty to terrify an anarchist. There was nothing that stood between Boone's kind and this free future but a few roving bands of savages. The man who had tortured to death the seventeen-year-old son of Daniel Boone had been a guest at Boone's table. What can you do with varmints like that? The day was to come when Boone with his own hands would cleanly kill the boy's murderer.

Now Dan's daughter was in the hands of another former guest of her father's, Hanging Maw, who spoke plenty English, as he looked over the flower he had torn from its soil.

Jemima squared her shoulders. 'I'm Dan Boone's daughter,' she said in a tone that meant, 'and you'll be sorry.'

'Are these your sisters?' demanded Hanging Maw.

'Yes,' said Jemima instantly, casting the cloak of her prestige over them.

Hanging Maw grinned appreciatively. 'If Boone comes after you,' he reasoned, as a snake does which can strike if you move and strike if you do not, 'we'll ambush him. If he catches up with you, we'll tomahawk you. So we have done pretty well for old Boone this time. Now begin to run, you girls. We have far to go. March!'

'I can't go,' said Jemima, gritting her teeth. 'I can't walk a step; my foot is hurt, and I haven't a shoe for it.'

'I have no shoes either,' said little Fanny stoutly.

Grimly in their leniency the Indians gave the two girls moccasins; it wasn't to death they were taking these captives.

The girls were young, but not too young to sense what was coming. They had only one hope — to delay their abduction, and no stratagem could be too foolish or too dangerous to try. For, once they were over the Ohio River, toward which the Indians were driving them, they would speedily be smelling the bitter smoke of Shawnee towns. So they snaggled their skirts on every thorn they brushed by, to slow their passage and leave a thread of trail. So their five big angry captors slashed their skirts off short. Betsy, who had heels to her shoes, dug them into the soft forest soil to mark her steps, till the Indians knocked the heels off. They drove the girls into a stream and made them run down it so the trail would be lost. Jemima said they could kill her then and there, but she couldn't go another step on that foot of hers. So Hanging Maw ordered the willful three mounted upon a stray pony the party came across, but as soon as they were seated, the girls fell off, screaming so that the edge of the forest should hear them. Their captors put them back on, and they fell off and screamed again. Even the Indians laughed; it was fun, at first, having girls fall in your arms and pushing and pulling them back up on the pony. But at any minute the 'Long Knives,' the white Kentuckians, might miss these squaw children. And the vengeance of Boone was already a legend.

So they made the girls run again. The three broke off twigs surreptitiously. Caught at this, 'We're so tired,' they fluted, 'we're just dragging ourselves along by the bushes.' Tomahawks were lifted suggestively, and flashed red in the sunset light.

Now the wilderness dark was coming down. Now the girls were far, and alone with the five savage men. Each was tied, sitting upright, against a tree, and in their bonds they twisted all night, their hearts beating against the thongs binding their breasts. The fireflies went everywhere through the forest; they were free to go where they pleased, but they had no homes to return to. The big barred owl stared at the embers of the campfire. 'Who cooks for you-all?' he barked to Jemima. Or perhaps he was asking the Indians, who would soon have three young slaves in their lodges, to grind the corn and carry the water, and do all their bidding, with heads bent down in shame and fear.

In story, the Indian captive is always rescued, the besieged fort is always relieved. But in fact, there is not a county in all America, I suppose, where some roof was not fired by an Indian brand, or men at their plowing were not pierced through the shoulders by an arrow flying out of the woods, or captives were not run off like this, never again to see home.

The girls weren't even missed till sundown on Sunday. And just as Boonesborough picked up their trail, the mocking darkness closed in. All that Boone could do was to wait for morning and listen to the rending howl of the timber wolves. The dew was still only gray; it was an icy slap on the thighs when Daniel Boone took up the trail. Behind him came the brothers and the three young lovers of the stolen girls, with their rifles clenched in whitening knuckles. This fight was now elemental as a contest between elk in the fall. Before the sun set again all of one party must be dead. The girls would be in the arms of the other.

The Long Knives saw everything the girls had meant them to see; every shred of petticoat was a flag in the forest. Every twig was a pointing arrow, every footprint a cry. These men knew what the Indians would do in a canebrake: they'd scatter, with their captives, like quail; they'd cross their own tracks. But the pursuers untangled this knot as if they had been hounds. The trail was twelve hours cold when they started, but when Dan came on the carcass of the buffalo the Indians killed, it was still warm. Now it was a slain snake he found, and it was still twitching. Then the smell of woodsmoke came to Dan's nose; and he put up a quick hand in warning.

'We'll fan out,' he told the boys in a whisper, 'and surround 'em. Don't fire till I signal, for God's sake. Then fire all at once. Every man of them must go down at the first volley, or they'll kill the girls.'

When he'd given the grim youngsters time to find ambush and take aim, he parted the leaves and surveyed a little hollow. There she was, with her face hidden in Betsy's lap, her woodtangled locks flung out in despair. The older girl had her arm around Fanny, and she was looking straight toward Daniel Boone. But even this child of the wilderness did not detect a motion in the leaves as he raised his rifle and drew a bead.

One Indian was gathering wood, one was blowing on the fire, two were cutting up the buffalo hump, and Hanging Maw was just lighting up the pipe of a man well content with what he has got. The crack of the rifles and a fountain of blood from an Indian's vein, right into Betsy's face, came together.

'That's Daddy!' shouted Jemima, on her feet in a flash.
'Run, gals, run!'

And they ran — from their dead and dying captors — laughing and sobbing, into the arms of their rescuers, and were kissed by lips stern with anger and fierce with happiness.

Betsy and her Sam were pronounced man and wife by Dan's brother Squire, who was a sort of lay preacher. Old Colonel Calloway wasn't too sure how legal that was, but the young folks meant their vows, and that's what counts. As for Fanny, she was told she was a minnow yet, and was thrown back in the creek. Flanders Calloway stoutly allowed to Dan that he'd won Mima for fair this time; Mima 'lowed it too. But Dan was firm; they'd have to wait till she was fifteen and a woman.

'Yes, sir,' said Dan Boone's daughter.

It all happened just that way, down to the bend of a twig, the shred of a petticoat! There's no man would tamper with facts so perfect, and Boone's story needs no luster from me. Jemima's story, of course, was no more than a frontier incident. But put together, those incidents, and the men and women who triumphed through them, have made our history.

Eastward, over the mountains, history was being written. While Hanging Maw had been lurking across the river from Boonesborough, the pen of Thomas Jefferson had been writing: *When in the course of human events, it becomes necessary for one people to dissolve the political bands which have connected them with another . . .*

The news of the Declaration of Independence flew fast, for those times; it was only two months in going three hundred wilderness miles to Boonesborough. Boone and the rest of the 'common people' of Transylvania turned and looked in each other's eyes. What's this? Look here! This Declaration says that all men are created free and equal, does it? Well, can you square that with what the Proprietors laid down for law? With monopoly in land grants? With quit-rents, and liveries of seisin? You can't — and they didn't want to. A man has certain inalienable rights, and that's a fact, sir!

So the feudalistic dream and scheme that was Transylvania

went up in smoke in the gigantic bonfire that Boonesborough lit to celebrate the Declaration of Independence. But though Transylvania never became a political state, it was — and is — a state of mind. There are a few who still dwell in it. But the rest of us have become the nation in which Harrodsburg, today a town of 4673, gave sixty-six of its boys — whether now living or dead no one knows, at this writing, **but the Japanese** — to the defense of Bataan.

11

Tall Men and Long Knives

I STARTED OUT TO WRITE this book for a man who may be dead and so could certainly never read it; I find I am also writing it for Heck, whom I know to be alive, as of yesterday. But it's more than possible that he won't read it either.

I shan't mind too much, because I could go to his house and say the same things. I could go to his office and — such is the fine old Spanish tempo of this town — sit on his desk and talk over world affairs in his business hours. There was never a man on earth so easy to get on with.

But I worry him, I can see, when he gets the mistaken idea that because he's a business man I mistrust his ideals. Bless you, no, Heck! That story about Henderson's land company didn't have you in it anywhere. I'm happy to say you make a good living out of real estate, but you don't believe in government of the people by the stockholders any more than Jim Harrod did. You believe in one of the most unattainable Utopias of all — as little government as possible. You and Jim Harrod have always liked to run your own affairs. Jim would have cared less for government by questionnaire than even you, for he couldn't read or write. But he dictated a mighty sharp protest to the Transylvania Company when it arbitrarily boosted the price of the public domain.

And when the Proprietors tried to put one of their number

into a seat in Congress, Harrodsburg held an election of its own. It sent to the Revolutionary legislature in Williamsburg a young fellow named Clark, George Rogers Clark. They thought a lot of him in Kentucky. He'd been raised up quite a scholar; he'd fought in Lord Dunmore's War, he'd surveyed all around here, and settled in at Harrodsburg among the first. Now he was one of them, the frontier men. They'd seen him fight, they'd seen him with an axe, they'd heard him laugh, that big, catching laugh of all the Clark family, they'd heard him talk when he meant what he said, and they trusted him to stand up for them down there in Williamsburg. So they sent him off the regular way, the way that Americans had begun to run things from the beginning, with no special privileges asked or granted. The Harrodsburg way, we'll call it, the opposite of the Transylvania way.

And I'm frank to say it's the Transylvanians that I do mistrust. You'll find them wherever you are. My carpenter told me how he had recently been ordered to come to a mansion in the suburbs here, to build basement cupboards three feet deep; the day he finished the job, trucks arrived at the back door and the servants unloaded boxes and barrels of food supplies and hustled them in to hide under lock and key. Whoever else might go without, it was not to be the Transylvanians in that house. That's putting the philosophy of that state in petty terms; but you can expand the same simple incident to world size, and where do you get?

Now the state of Transylvania has been set up many a time since, under other names. There have been men in the United States Senate who represented the stockholders and not the people. Some cities, some districts, have been practically in the bag for the stockholders for long periods. There were men, you remember, at the Constitutional Convention who thought that the primary purpose of government is to protect the rich. Not so long ago, even a President opined that 'the business of America is business.'

Harrodsburgers say that the business of America is a

better America, and they'd agree with you, Heck, that in that happy land a man's personal business too would flourish. Abroad, we've had the reputation of being, all of us, Transylvanians. That's perhaps because enterprise and energy are traits of the Transylvanian, just as much as his belief that it's self-interest that makes the world go round, as Henderson told the House of Delegates under the great old elm. We know the foreigner's picture of us doesn't wholly square with the facts, but we must have given him the impression somehow. The truth is that Transylvania and Harrodsburg have been with us from the beginning, as once there were both Bethlehem and Rome. There's not one of our little towns, I suppose, without some of both in it. Not Marblehead, not Fredericksburg, not my town.

So I'm not idealizing Harrodsburg, and when I take its name to stand for all that an American town ought to be, I'm not saying that everybody in Harrodsburg is as good as the best of its citizens; to tell the truth, I don't know a soul in the town. I went there because a native said I mustn't miss it; she was a girl I met at Berea College, and she'd probably never been anywhere but Harrodsburg. But you are not necessarily mistaken because you are naïve. And I saw that what she was so proud of was what we are all proud of, wherever we live.

So for a little while I had the privilege, so highly recommended by Stevenson, of being a stranger there myself. This has certain great advantages over having the knowing show you the town. If you don't ask the town for the special favors offered an announced guest, it doesn't put on any company manners.

It was two or three weeks after the fall of Bataan that we drove into Harrodsburg. The place was just going about its business, as it did within the old stockade even when the Shawnees had run off some of its boys. It's a perfectly ordinary town, except for the fort. What you try to picture, among the lonely violets of Boonesborough, you can see for yourself at Harrodsburg. They have carefully put back as much of their youth as they could. There is the stockade, built around a spring, and the cabins built within the stockade; the school is there, with its log benches and deerhide map; the blockhouses hold the corners squarely, and within their hard male protection lie the little hearths and the women things that belong to them. Ann McGirty's spinning-wheel is there; she was a famous spinner and weaver, and if Homer had written the epic of Kentucky, he would have made Minerva jealous of her. Hers was the first little wheel to turn in all this western wilderness; the thread she spun on it out of buffalo hair has become a rope so strong that whatever the Japanese may have done to those sixty-six boys cannot have frayed it.

You feel confident of that when you look into the little log rooms where Harrodsburg men were first born. You might call what you see there squalor; you might call it glory. They didn't have what you and I would need; but what they had they made do for plenty. There are Mark McGohon's sword that he carried in the Revolution and would use again in the War of 1812, and his bride Betsy's corded cherry bed, brought over the mountains, with her hand-woven 'kivers' for on top and a trundle bed to go under it that the two of them would presently fill. Mark had his rifle-gun, and Betsy had her firebox in which she could fetch coals from a neighbor's when her own hearth-fire went out. The turkey-wing broom kept the hearth neat, and she had a board to make johnnycake on, if she had meal, salt, and water. All the way from the East came her pewter spoons and her bits of china, not broken even yet, her bean pot and trivet, her spiders and andirons and her rocker. She had her English clock to tick out time that had never been kept before, and she had her tallow candle, her candlestick and night-stand, to hollow out of the wilderness dark a small brave shrine of human light.

You can find, too, in the fort, the text for all our Harrodsburgs. A frontier preacher chose it from Exodus 23:30:

'*By little and little I will drive them out from before thee until thou be increased and inherit the land.*'

Boonesborough, St. Asaph's, Logan's Station, Bryan's Station, Boiling Springs — they were like to Harrodsburg as seeds in a pod are alike, seeds that we scattered apart in the woods as we came advancing. But it was long before the Yellow Boys were driven out from before us. They too had their home fires, their blooded knives, their smoke-blacked kettles. They gave ground hardly.

Jemima Boone Calloway would have been a bride of a few months or perhaps only a few days when the Shawnees hurled the hatchet at the log gates of Boonesborough. They were led by Mkahdaywahmayquah; Boone, who knew him well, understandably preferred to call him Blackfish. And Blackfish, like forked lightning, was striking everywhere at once. He was at Harrodsburg; he was at McClelland's Station; he was at every cabin in the woods. He was at Boonesborough, and with all the other settlements under siege, he prepared to finish off his deadliest enemy.

Jemima knew what was in the wind, because the cows had stood in the clearing that morning, when she drove them out of the fort, snuffing the air and switching unhappy tails. A cow could smell an Indian, it seems, and hated the smell with all its bucolic heart. The boy of the charmed life, Simon Kenton, Dan's right-hand man, saw an Indian dash from the woods and tomahawk a Boonesborough citizen within sixty yards of the fort; he ran for his rifle and shot the enemy as he was lifting the white man's hair. The shot brought Boone and a dozen others pouring out of the fort. Kenton saw another Indian draw a bead on Daniel, but Simon did not let the red finger squeeze the trigger. In a moment the woods emptied out Shawnees as a kicked anthill spills ants. Daniel was down, with a bullet in his ankle, and Simon, his powder spent, was standing over him clubbing the Indians with his rifle butt as they came. The women of Boonesborough were watching from the stockade; they saw their heroes falling, but suddenly the gate was flung open and out dashed Jemima to her daddy. With Simon's help Dan Boone's daughter dragged him back inside the stockade. We are what we are, you see, because we raise up the same kind after us.

Firing the crops, running off the cattle, Blackfish let his lightning strike and kill and strike in another place. He wasn't ready yet to carry on the great sieges he was planning, with Boonesborough for chief prize. But he left his foes dead and mutilated at the very walls of each Kentucky fort. While Burgoyne and Cornwallis were countermarching against Washington on the other side of the mountains, the Shawnees, with arms provided by the British from Canada, were harrying our western frontier. If they had broken through the defenses of Boone and Harrod and Logan and Bryan and McClelland, they would have been on the backs of Virginia, Pennsylvania, and New York.

While he was getting salt for his settlement at the Salt Licks, Boone was captured by Blackfish, and held for six months in captivity. Old Blackfish admired his enemy so intensely that he declared Daniel his adopted son; they named him Sheltowee, Wide Mouth, and the simple savage became convinced that Boone had now perceived the delights and perquisites of being a Shawnee and would never try to escape. But all great Indian-fighters have been great diplomatists too. They knew — and it took a good part of a lifetime to learn it — what an Indian was thinking and what he would then do, as well as the Indian knew about the instincts and wary actions of the deer he stalked. So versed, Wide Mouth outwitted his dear foster parents and brothers-in-the-tribe completely.

Covering a hundred and sixty miles on foot in four days, Dan Boone got back to Boonesborough just ahead of Blackfish's surprise attack on it, of which Dan carried the warning. Though Rebecca, having given up her husband for dead this time, had gone back to North Carolina, Mima was there to fling her arms around him, and Flanders to pump his hand. And young Kenton, vigilant in the woods as a crow on a dead tree-top, came flying back to the fort, just ahead of Blackfish, with the news that George Rogers Clark had led Harrodsburg clean to the Mississippi and whipped the British at Kaskaskia in Illinois.

Now a tingle ran through the autumn air; now the woods began to hang out their battle flags among maple and tulip poplar and red oak and black. Behind that forest screen gathered the Indians, painted for war — four hundred of them, Shawnees under Blackfish, Wyandots and Ottawas, Blackbird the Chippewa, old Moluntha the harrier, Catebeccas, who had lifted scalps long ago at Braddock's defeat. They were well armed, and by white hands; Governor Hamilton of Ontario, 'the Hair-Buyer,' as the angry Americans called him, had made them a present of a hundred and fifty dozen scalping knives, and eighty pounds of red paint to daub on their faces for battle, and powder and lead enough to bring to its knees a fort ten times as strong as Boonesborough.

But even an Indian would prefer to get what he wanted by palaver rather than by blood his side, too, might spill. So Blackfish offered to parley, not without sincere reproaches to his ungrateful 'son' for so privately and hastily departing from the bosom of his Shawnee family. Boone spun out the negotiations. He twirled them as fine and as long as a hair from Jemima's head. For every day gained meant that the letter he had dispatched to Virginia for help was jogging farther eastward over the Wilderness Trail.

Every day the red and the gold and the russet patched more brightly the forest walls; the soft air grew sharper at morning and evening; the tension grew. On Boonesborough's ramparts, behind the stockade, its women, even the black slaves, paraded with muskets hour after hour; they were dressed in men's clothing, and they held up their heads and squared their shoulders and looked as boldly male as they were bravely woman. Outside the fort the parley droned on.

Every night the cattle came plodding in to the door of the stockade, and every morning were driven out to pasture again. The Indians let the herd go through their lines, tolerantly sure that before long the beasts would be galloping before them, driven as the women and children would be driven, toward the Shawnee towns over the Ohio. And every day the tense-cheeked women within the fort sent out, to those of their men who were negotiating, a feast of assertive plenty, to show the red chiefs how abundantly Boonesborough was stocked for a siege. The fact of it was that they stood close to the edge of starvation. As for water, they never yet had dug that well.

In the midst of the parley, Blackfish tried treachery. There were a few touch-and-go minutes when each white negotiator was under a pile of attacking Indians. Then the rifles blazed from the stockade, and the savages were running for the forest cover.

Next it was fire that Blackfish tried. He rolled flaming bales of flax to the stockade's log walls; he hurled firebrands on the cabin roofs. It took every drop of water remaining in Boonesborough to put out the last blaze.

And then, while Jemima and her kind were running bullets, while the very children were clawing at the earth to get that well finished, Blackfish began to tunnel. From the bank of the Kentucky he started digging; his tunnel was aimed to go straight under the walls of the fort.

Boone countermined. The opposing forces each would hear, under the ground, the enemy's pick and shovel working. Boonesborough taunted the Shawnee. 'Going to blow you plumb to hell!' it cheerfully promised. The Indians said less, but shot more; from the hill above the fort their sharpshooters had the compound within range. So Boonesborough unhinged its cabin doors and, carrying them for shields on their backs, men moved about in squads under Shawnee fire.

Even the sky was holding its breath. There wasn't food or ammunition or water enough for two more days of life in the little log citadel. Then in the night the clouds broke and a storm fell through, a blotting and riotous darkness that offered perfect cover for attack. Now they would be coming; now they must be there, right out there, in the black and the lashing rain. The sky split in flashes, and Boonesborough's sentinels strained to see the first naked red leg flung over the stockade, the first running invader within. Nothing yet, and the blackness and rain wiped out that chance to see, and there was only waiting left, crowded with thunder and pounding of the blood and those thoughts that break through a man's wall against them and get to his heart. Thoughts of the scalping and burning to come, and the women run off, to be lost in a long dark slavery.

All night the autumn rain stormed, and the Indians did not come. Instead it was day that came, slowly, fearfully over the looming woods, a thin silvery light that trembled down every dripping leaf. The raindrops glistened on spiderwebs that stretched unbroken from twig to weed, frail fences that had held through the long night. There was no footprint marring the sheen on the wet prostrate grasses. There was no clamor of crows in the brightening sky; only, high on a barefingered hickory tree, were two black gossips mocking and chattering in crow talk, as they will do when they know there is no one about. There was no smell of roasting meat from the woods, nothing but the shadowy reek of toadstools, and no smoke but the aimless smoking of dank ground along the river.

The men and women of Boonesborough looked up at the pole they had raised when they raised their walls, and saw a high-hearted morning breeze lift out of the folds of the flag. Theirs was the first American flag that ever flew beyond the mountains, the old flag, so like ours of today but with the thirteen stars in a wreath. Such a little flag, such a big one!

Then they looked long at the woods again, and at last Daniel said it. If he said they were gone, they were gone.

So the storm in the night that could have cloaked attack

had been used by the Shawnees to cover their retreat. They had got a bear by the tail, and were glad of a chance to let go safely. Boonesborough now took stock of its losses. Not a man had been killed, though many wounded. Not a woman was hurt, except for Jemima Calloway, and the bullet that pinked her had merely glanced into her soft little buttock; a twitch of her skirt fetched it out.

Now the sun from the rim of the world shot its long lances to catch the forest tree-tops. It rose, and the light stole down the branches, down the boles. It flooded all Kentucky; it gave back the colors and the shapes of things. And lo! it was the morning of the eighth day; it was everyday again, and Boonesborough looked on it and found it good.

The men of Logan's Station had marched to the aid of Boonesborough at the first alarm; they'd been shut up in the fort all through the siege with no one in their own settlement but boys to guard the women. They swallowed their breakfast in a gulp, and set out to learn what was left of their own. That very morning some girls outside Logan's Station saw a column of men running toward their settlement. 'It's Indians!' they called, and they turned and ran for the fort. But one, braver or scareder than the rest, looked back. 'Lor' God!' she said devoutly. 'It's our own boys!'

You can read in the history books how Clark and his Kentuckians carried the war to Vincennes, how they captured old Hamilton the Hair-Buyer and brought him back to Virginia. Nobody touched him as he was led across Kentucky; he passed unmolested through Craborchard and Hazelpatch, over Dreaming Creek and Troublesome, through the Gap and back over the Wilderness Road, through the Shenandoah and down to Tidewater. But in the courtyard of the Governor's Palace at Williamsburg, Governor Thomas Jefferson let him wait four hours on his horse in the rain. And by Hamilton's piteous account of it, he was punished on his most punishable parts — his dignity.

But history wasn't through with Kentucky. Long after

Cornwallis had surrendered, the Shawnees were still on the warpath. No other part of the country suffered in the Revolution as Kentucky did, for they were fighting enemies who were not Christians. It's bad enough when Christians fight each other, but there is no horror like that of being in the power of those who despise compassion and have with them no God on whom you can call.

And no other people put so much of their manpower into the field as Kentucky's. Indeed, they had no army; they were all civilians, but all fighters. In the War of 1812 Kentucky put five times her quota under arms; in the Revolution she paid a terrible price for her independence. That was because she staked everything, again and again. Over and over Harrod and Clark, Boone and Logan, were out on the offensive; they had to leave cabins and stations unguarded, to strike the enemy before he could strike. Once they met with ambush and defeat; that was at the battle of Blue Licks. Boone carried his dead son's body off that battlefield. There was hardly a family on the frontier that did not weep the loss of a protector after Blue Licks. But Clark gathered up all the scattered ranks; again he crossed the Ohio, and this time he burned the Shawnee towns, and now it was the Indian women who wailed, and their children who hid in hollow trees.

Later Wayne would come, Mad Anthony, to strike red hip and thigh at Fallen Timbers. Then William Henry Harrison, to break the power of the greatest confederacy and uprising in all Indian history, at Tippecanoe.

Somewhere in all this border fighting, we've lost track of Colonel Henderson. Colonel he was, but I haven't found the record of his deeds in the Revolution. Sometimes he's heard of, lobbying in Williamsburg, and sometimes he swims with bigger fish wherever the fugitive Continental Congress was convening. I'm not saying he didn't do what a good Transylvanian should — look after the interests of the investors. Perhaps, as president of the company, he was supposed to stay with his ship. I only know that he wasn't in Kentucky all during these flaming years.

Boonesborough had forgotten about Henderson too. It took a long time to unsnaggle the worthless claims that men had piled up in the slapjack of the boom. For a few years Boonesborough, a terminus of the Wilderness Trail, flourished as an outfitting place for those advancing the frontier even farther. But Boone left it to found Boone's Station, a little way off. Not all its memories were good ones to Daniel; he'd been sold here, and he was minded to write on a clean slate. With his going departed the glory. In a few years there was not a cabin standing in Boonesborough. Uniquely among the towns I choose, this one goes back to the grass.

And Jemima? The Lord looked on her and blessed her. Her children were John and James and Larkin — three boys — and her five girls, Sarah, Frances, Elizabeth, Susannah, and Minerva. She raised them all, and they all married. Her daughter Sarah, for instance, was married to James Barnes, and he begat James and John and Larkin, and William and Calloway and Flanders (who married Obedience Grigg) and Lilburn and Volney and Andrew — nine boys; and now for the names of her girls, Rhoda and Jemima and Minerva and Margaret and Hulda and Cynthia and Elizabeth, and six more I've forgotten.

So Jemima the First had seventy-two grandchildren. Indeed, old Daniel Boone had an estimated four hundred great-grandchildren, of whom, however, he lived to know or hear of only about a hundred. *By little and little I will drive them out from before thee until thou be increased and inherit the land.*

Kentucky, the child of Virginia and North Carolina, became the mother of Missouri, southern Illinois, southern Indiana. The finest volunteers on the Lewis and Clark expedition were the Kentucky men. Kentuckians became, by growing just a little taller in their boots, the Mountain Men of the Rockies. Kit Carson was born near Boonesborough in 1809. In that same year, near Harrodsburg, was born Abraham Lincoln.

12

Portrait on My Wall

THIS IS ONE OF THOSE days when the morning opened like an invitation. From my pillow I see the first ruddy sunlight touch the opposite climbing height of the canyon, wash the night out of the hollows, burnish the chaparral, brighten to joy the clear blue above the Coast Range skyline.

Then, in the times that were, not so long ago, I would turn my head and look in my wife's eyes, see there my own lighthearted hunger for the road, and say, 'Let's!' No need to explain to her why I suddenly wanted to go, or tell her what to pack. She knew the formula: take clothes for hot and cold running weather. What I took was maps and binoculars, bird guides and plant manuals; with as brief preparation as possible we got in the car and let her roll. Quietly at first, downhill by the long streets bordered with olives and eucalyptus, then at a clip when we struck the highway; and the sea, sending its glittering endless frontal attack to crash and crash on the shore beside us, blew away the drowsy perfume of the citrus orchards. Soon what we smelled, before we could smell it, was Nevada sagebrush, the piñon smoke of New Mexican chimneys, the rain falling resinous from Colorado spruce and Oregon fir and the frondy arbor vitae, giant canoe cedar, that grows all the way up into Alaska.

If school was keeping, we parked the three boys there. If

not, we scooped them up as we left. They never knew when we'd be going, but they knew how to behave. They are trained to be quiet from the start, to sing as the day grows long and they tire, really to see what they look at, never to read aloud from billboards or comment crossly on traffic, or even to ask where we are going. For often we would not know, till we were on our way. Our chief rule for ourselves was simply to get started. If you wait a day, you'll wait a week; if you wait a week, you'll stay at home, we said blithely.

It was carefree, it was headlong, it was often financially reckless. More than once I've taken my last cash out of the bank, to buy me another fresh slice of America. And the worst, as well as the best, of working for yourself is that there's no other boss to tell you that you've got to stay home with your nose to the grindstone. I could always retort to myself that Nature was my immediate business, and I had to do some field work, didn't I?

Well, the treasure I got for my money I can take with me, tax-free, as long as I live, maybe longer. It's what I came west to get, like any Forty-Niner. I had known my Middle West and the South and the eastern seaboard; I had tasted winy New Hampshire Augusts, and followed the haunting skyline of the Blue Ridge. I had sailed all the Great Lakes but Ontario, and been to the tip of Florida; I knew the Mississippi right down to the delta, and had studied the depth of the prairie loam. So I came west, to find Pike's Peak like a white tidal wave sweeping onto the plains, and see if trees could grow as tall as the redwoods they told of, and throw my lasso over the snowy truncated cones of Mount Rainier, Mount Hood, Mount St. Helens. I came here to live just so as to have such neighbors. And any day that I dared, I could set forth to see them. Any day when I woke in the morning and felt sweeping over me a tingling nostalgia for my country, three thousand miles of it, from coast to coast.

Today was a day like that. It opened as glistening fresh as a split fruit. I got up at a workaday pace; why hurry? I wasn't going anywhere, without rubber or gas. Before the day's labor took me, I stepped out to breathe the morning and to see the world from my foothold in it. There lay my town below; the streets went spreading away and, in the countryside beyond, the roads looped over the hills and out of sight. There was little moving on them; the town looked toylike, innocently vulnerable. High above, a deep thrum filled the sky, like bees in a vast blue corolla. Upon that note our times are pitched; the world over, we vibrate to it in terror or rejoicing. Now the Marines passed over, glinting in echelon. Those are the men that are going places.

I turned and went into my study, to settle at this desk. It's still the only place I'm useful, and that chiefly to my family and myself. Uncle Sam isn't so hard up yet that he needs to try to make a soldier out of the likes of me, and there appears to be almost nothing that I can do for my fellow men who are soldiers. I found this out when I was asked to speak in a church the other night; my topic was the peace that we expect to bring about by this war. I know that I don't know anything about this subject, but nobody knows about it. Oh, there are plenty of people who can tell you what the peace ought to be like, but as almost no two are in accord, and only one at the most could be quite right, it follows that all the others — no matter what the circulation of the paper they write for, or whose private secretary they were at the League of Nations, or how popular they are with women's clubs — must be more or less wrong. Nevertheless, the more we discuss it the better, and that Sunday night I chipped in my two cents' worth. For the peace will be what you and I are prepared to think it and make it. God, they say, inspired the Bible, but the world we live in is as good as our behavior. So the noblest peace will not last if we do not underwrite it.

Well, I sounded off on this note, and they listened with more respect than I'm used to, because I was talking from a pulpit. It was a slightly disillusioning experience to me to find out how easy this is. An isolated and scientific part of myself was astounded to hear my more public personality referring to the will of God precisely as though it had been made known to me. And the pulpit looks different seen from behind; there were all sorts of little buzzers and light-switches right under my omnipotent hand, and the place was wired up for loud-speaking, as from Sinai. So I'm afraid I let myself go about brotherly love.

I know I begged my audience not to make this a race war. I said I'd heard an army major growling on the radio that we'd lose if we didn't all of us hate a lot more bitterly. I took advantage of this sanctuary within the church to defy the major. I said that hate is a lethal weapon; ignorant civilians are not supposed to brandish it or the first thing they know they'll wound a lot of innocent people. However, even civilians can learn to shoot; they can in time learn to hate. But it is very difficult to unlearn that lesson. And if, I said, by the time we got to the peace, we had nothing but hate for the peoples we must conquer, then we could not keep that peace.

Now I'm proud to hate certain ideas, but I am ashamed of myself when I hate peoples. Some take just the other way; they find it easiest to hate individuals or nations or races, but they do not want to be bothered to inspect an idea and have a resultant passion about it. I couldn't, in church that night, know who was agreeing with me, because speakers are not applauded in the house of God, but as I slunk down the side steps — I really couldn't make a recessional through the back of the chancel, you know — I was intercepted by a concerned young sailor.

'That's all right,' he blurted, 'what you said about having to live on one planet together when it's over, but how's a man going to kill other men without hating their guts?'

And I answered him not, neither did I know what to say.

We agreed, when I could find my tongue, that war is a monstrous immorality. It is right to fight, but wrong to start the fight; that much is easy. But war violates personal and national morality, even while drawing it to its greatest height.

The only good thing in it — and of course its moral beauty towers and glitters — is that the lives laid down in it are given for love. Hate is but one of the wounds the enemy inflicts on us.

It's not exactly a new thing to say, but it is a true thing and worthy to be received of all men, that a nationalist is one who hates all foreigners, more or less — you'll usually find him hating a lot of people inside his own borders too — while a patriot is a man who loves his country. So he can understand why men in other countries love theirs.

As you've guessed, I only thought of most of this on the way home from the church. The sailor rejoined his battlewagon innocent of these pronouncements, and I rejoined the arms of my family, a man of peace not yet found worthy of real sacrifices.

That's all a digression, and a confession, to say why I fall silent around men in uniform. Oh, not around superior officers; they won't have to use a bayonet; they're crammed full of certainties and more than ready to voice them. They take almost professionally gloomy and cynical views of the peace, as perhaps good military men should. I'm inclined to talk back to them; why not? since where we're going nobody has been. But I can't do anything for a younger man, for a boy torn from bosomy Georgia, or a farm on the Sangamon, or the pavements of Evansville, Indiana. And I wince when they thank me for buying them a drink or taking them home to dinner. My wife seems to have the hang of it better; when that handsome Marine thanked her yesterday, she cordially told him, 'Oh, you know that you give civilian women a thrill.' Answered he, in the gallant accents of Alabama, 'Lady, it's us get a thrill from civilian women.'

It's a relief, when I've been mulling ideas too big for me, to get up and knock out my pipe in the fireplace, throw on another log, and dig into my tobacco jar. And on these small peripatetic travels around my study, which are the limit of today's excursion, I bump into all of America. For on my wall I have hung a picture. Familiar as it is, I cannot grow tired of looking at it, any more than a man could grow tired of his mother's face. You might call it a portrait, of greatness. It's a chart, too, of a mighty and unfinished adventure. It's a grand, over-all view of home, yours and mine — a map of America.

Any way I study it, that map is inexhaustible. Sometimes it looks to me like a living organism, with venous and arterial river systems, and a muscular armature of highways and railroads pulling and distributing weight, every city a nervous plexus connected by floss-fine lines of communication. When I see it that way, I think of the pulsing life-blood flowing through this country, and remember how the trains go tearing off the miles with a soft scream of ripping distance, that echoes in the mountain passes. Of how the boats hoot where the rivers curve between high bluffs, and of the laborious puff of engines shunting freight around crowded yards. Of the wind making a compass of the beach grass on Plum Island off Ipswich, and whipping up the wavelets in Marblehead harbor so that the boys' catboats chuckle as they tramp them down. Sometimes when you stand on a jutting rock in the Craggies, you can hear our American wind pluck up all the Appalachian forest like strings and cry our anthem. And all across the prairies you can see it run ahead of you, stamping this way and that like a ghostly herd. We have strung Kansas like a harp, with barbed-wire fences and telegraph lines, and the wind makes a hollow music in them there; it tears the frills off your thinking, slaps you on the back, whistles like a rain of arrows past your ears. If you do not like wind, you will not like Kansas, and if you do not like Kansas high plains, you will not like the West. Not really, however much you enjoy the famous scenery of Rockies or Sierra.

Then Colorado, the hard male breast of it slowly lifting with a breath of pride. Beef now, not hogs and wheat. Buttes and mesas, the land rising thus the better to see across distance. An endless convoy of clouds across the rim of earth, and pilot hawks quartering for prey. Cactus and tumbleweed and yucca, signs of a grand carelessness of what we call useful in the land. And then the scudding low white clouds that are not clouds, but snow on the vanguard of the Rockies.

The stem of my pipe traveling the map searches that continental backbone and stops a moment. That's the Lemhi Pass, right there, and I came over it on foot, following Lewis and Clark, that summer we picked up their trail at the Three Forks in Montana and went with them all down the gorge of the Columbia to their campsite at Clatsop in Oregonian woods. I called it field work, of course, but it was holiday of the highest. The oldest of my boys, at least, is on to me now; he was along on that trip, and one evening when we stopped for the night in a cottage on Oregon rocks, he looked out of the surf-sprayed window dreamily at the Pacific and murmured, 'What fun we'll have when Father decides he must follow the footsteps of Magellan!'

In those years it was always wilderness I was hunting. I thirsted for it as if it were medicine for the ills of our soul-sick people; I talked that way too; and there's something in it. We suffer from our success in overmastering Nature; our population centers are crowded to morbidity; our interdependence makes most of us specialists incapable of surviving outside a narrow field. An environment so delicately adjusted to keep humans in undreamed-of comfort and distracting pleasure is more vulnerable than a stockaded frontier settlement.

Wilderness, if we could have it back, would bring no end to poverty and starvation and maladjustment. But what we have left of it — and that is not two per cent of the total area of the country, preserved by government agencies — is a necessity, I think, to our national health. Increasingly, in the pre-war years, the American people have sought their wilderness areas. You'd meet those vigorous citizens, singly or in twos or companies, starting off for the high places, the open spaces, the tall timber and the deep water. How full of anticipation they looked as they set forth, portaging canoes, cinching their pack-animals, with city whiteness still upon them! How bronzed and wind-flecked they were when you saw them scrambling down the trails to civilization again!

For a week or a month, or three, you might see the flash of their paddles on the waters of northern Maine, the curl of their campfire smoke joining the dreamy haze of the Nantahalas, and the shining of their tents in the Adirondacks. They'd wave to you from trout brooks of western Montana, and you found them on the High Sierra in California, chock full of proud new lore of cirques and escarpments and rock flowers and the nesting of rare alpine finches.

Our Nature was our mother, and her children still turn back to her. For three hundred years in American history, wilderness was a prime factor. It was the enemy then, but it made the characters of the men and women who fought it. Its bracing influence washed far back, like a fresh wind, into the settled life of the old Atlantic seaboard communities. Emerson's essay on 'Self-Reliance' has been called the piece of writing most influential on American life of the last century ever written by an American. And it is typical frontier philosophy.

Our political sentiments have always been influenced by that philosophy. Jefferson, though never a frontier man, was carried into and kept in the presidency by the frontier votes, because he was wilderness-minded. For the same reason, he bought, over the misgivings of many, all Louisiana, doubling the size of the United States, and then sent Lewis and Clark to extend the meaning of 'Louisiana' to include Idaho, Oregon, and Washington. Andrew Jackson and William Henry Harrison were wilderness presidents too, with the frontier vote behind them. Their tradition was strong enough to help sweep Abe Lincoln into office. The public and Teddy both preferred to think of Theodore Roosevelt not as a New York Dutch aristocrat, but as the 'Rough Rider' out of the West, who rode up Pennsylvania Avenue yipping and swinging his lariat, into the White House. The wilderness is our longest saga and the greatest of all our true legends. For in the beginning it taught the men and women who fought it that they were the people who couldn't be licked. And so we are still believing that of ourselves.

Only in the heroic past of our country, you'd say, only on the red man's side of the vanished frontier, could there be hundreds of square miles of centuries-old, virgin forest. Only in the dreams of Daniel Boone in his grave could antlered elk walk free and proud and friendly. But, in what I must reverently call God's good time, I got there. I stood in a forest so deep and vast that its beauty was dreadful. The crowns of the trees interlocked till they shut out the sky. Their trunks stood so close that they made walls around us. The deep surging sound of the wind in the boughs was utter loneliness, and in the long gloom of that place you heard how mortal was your own breathing. My wife and I looked in one another's eyes, each to see if into the other the same awe had entered. The children, who usually romp and shout when set free of the car, could not find their voices. Only, the youngest drew in a deep breath and let it out in a sigh — the sigh of human humility that you will hear from the lips of those who have been thinking too long about the stars and the spaces between them.

We were in a stand of timber covering an almost uninhabited area the size of the state of Connecticut. The Olympic Peninsula, which is in the extreme northwest corner of the United States, exhibits this great difference from the Nutmeg State — that whereas there are about three hundred and thirty-three persons living on every square mile, on the average, of Connecticut's land area, the Olympic Peninsula is populated by an average of from one to eight persons to the square mile — and most of those are concentrated along the lone highway that winds about its salty margin. Only imagine a Connecticut dominated by a range of mountains running up to eight thousand feet, capped with everlasting snow. A Connecticut covered from sea-level to timberline with an unbroken forest, principally coniferous, whose roots interlock as solidly as those of grass in heavy turf, whose canopy crosses, a hundred feet and more above the ground, in a weave so close the light is dusky green below it, and the deep bog moss stretches from the foot of one tree to the next, like spider webs in a dungeon cellar, for miles and miles and miles.

The Olympic Mountains themselves are not easily visible from the solitary highway that encircles the Peninsula. They are deep in the interior, and hidden by forest-crowned, nearby hills. They are apt to be veiled, even at angles from which they might be visible, in rolling cloud caps, in trailing mists. They are consequently there and yet not there, for the traveler. You feel their presence; you know it by the white icy streams that come clattering down through the firs and spruces and hemlocks; only a great snowfield high in the center of the province could send down water of that clarity and temperature, in the dry season, with such perpetual and even flow.

But sometimes, topping a rise, peering up a long valley or through a pass, you get glimpses to stop the breath, of a high-tossed complex of peaks, like a leaping of great earth waves cresting in white. Sheerly, purely, those summits gleam at you, unattainable and lost again at a closure of the clouds or the turning of the road. Of all mountain ranges in the country, the Olympics have been least often seen, and remain the most mysterious. Their ultimate forests of alpine fir and white pine, mountain hemlock and Rocky Mountain juniper and Baker cypress — so different in component species from the lowland forests — are visible only as a far-off band of green beneath the snowcaps; only the bold and hardy ever breathe their spicy air.

And, in their own way, the Olympics are higher than our other mountains. That is, one sees them, when one sees them, from sea-level, and consequently every inch of their eight thousand feet is visibly height. Not even old Pike beats this, seen as it is from altitudes of six thousand. There is no mountain view in America more superb than that backward look, when your ferry stands off for Vancouver Island across the Straits of Juan de Fuca, at the congested might of the Olympics, with their feet in primeval forest and their white heads in the clouds.

The Olympic Peninsula may be wilderness gone to heaven, but in its wealth and no less in its health and emptiness, it is of a piece with the great wilderness which our ancestors found when they first came here. In the course of three centuries, the resources of American Nature made American people rich. Only with the opening of the present century did we come within sight of the end of what congressmen, sawing their arms and fluttering their hands, liked to read into the record as 'our boundless resources.'

But though not boundless, the wilderness had done its great work on American character. Primeval hardships leveled all men; so we became confirmed in democracy, changing it from a strange new theory to the common way of life. The great loneliness gave us the national trait of fraternalism. That's why Americans don't put forbidding hedges around their front lawns; exclusively high hedges are bad manners on Main Street, and suggest hard hearts or stuffed shirts. And the man on the pavement likes to believe that the man behind a hedge is missing more than he shuts out.

We call the wilderness ways of hospitality, inventiveness, hopefulness, and classlessness 'typically American.' If they are, they were born in us, and wilderness only brought them out. We remember that our pioneer ancestors may have made mistaken decisions, but they never died of indecision; they may have been narrow but they were seldom shallow, and what they lacked in knowledge they made up for in know-how. They started into the wilderness from the east with only thirteen stars in their banner. Now we've got forty-eight, and we're not stopping just because we've gone so far west that we've got east again.

How far we've gone everybody knows, by the daily paper

and the radio. Every day now it comes closer to home that the boys from Sweetwater and Bozeman and Uvalde are out in the wilderness again. God knows that Harrodsburg understands that now. And Emporia, Kansas. This is the town where Main Street grows wide as the world; William Allen White, the editor of Emporia's paper, has made his town somehow mean all American towns; he did this not by raising his voice but by being himself and letting Emporia stand forth as itself.

It's as simple as that, I suspect — America's rôle in the future of the world.

I should have liked, when I passed through Emporia on my last east-west journey, to go to his door and ask to look at him, this common-sense genius. I reflected, though, that he had better things to do and, being a writer myself, I paid him a more acceptable tribute — I walked into an Emporia bookstore and bought his *Forty Years on Main Street*. But I had also to pay a visit to the telegraph office, and there I saw a poster; it showed the silhouette of Australia. The shape of that continent is familiar now as a symbol of the farthest off in all the world, the most improbable land toward which the sunflower would ever turn. I asked the woman at the desk whether many people in this town had come in to take advantage of the special rates that the poster offered. 'You'd be surprised,' she answered, and she nodded her head toward the little antipodean continent as though it were no farther off than the state college that used to take the boys from home. 'We've got a stake in that place now,' she said.

Yes, Emporia has a stake in Australia, in China, in France, in Moscow, but God knows they've got a stake in Emporia too. If they haven't heard of it by name, they're thinking about it all the same. That map of America up on my wall may well look, to others as well as ourselves, like the biggest clearing in the wilderness.

The ocean is a wilderness, a great, briny, heaving and yawning waste. (And they're making sailors out of men from

Coeur d'Alene, these days.) The sky is a wilderness, windswept and limitless, treacherous and more dangerous than the sea. (And they're making flyers out of cowboys.) The African desert and the Papuan jungles are wilderness (and they've got Gloucester fishermen fighting in them). But nowhere on the globe is there wilderness like the thinking of our present enemies, in which there are no compass points of good and evil. It is this that I hate. It is this we must fight, long after the killing of men is done with. For that black jungle has deep roots, long suckers; it can come creeping back, yes, even into the clearing.

13

Utopia on the Wabash

THE WIDE EMPTINESS that was early American has always looked to Europeans like an unwritten page. Europe resembles one of our great-grandmother's letters, written across and then turned sidewise and crossed again, for economy of paper. Indeed it has been interlined and crossed out and written over, until there is no reading it. So that anyone in Europe who had a new proposition he wished to expound must get a new sheet to write on. And looking the world over, he usually found that this continent of ours was most nearly worthy of receiving his idea.

Our own Puritan ancestors, the first to found a permanent colony in this country, came with just such a notion of starting something new in a new place. And while it is not remotely true that our nation stems straight from Plymouth Rock, still their example and their success emboldened legions. It would be impossible even to catalogue all the movements, all the idealists, all the special pleaders who have come to America to save not only themselves but the world. These people may not have formed an actual majority over the simpler immigrants, but the color of their minds has certainly tinctured the national thinking. You may find the hue in wise men and in fools. It was this belief — that here we could make a better society, that here we could form a more perfect union — which gave us the Declaration of Independence and the Constitution. Washington, Jefferson, Lincoln, Emerson, Franklin D. Roosevelt — to mention but some of the wise — have all been native-born American idealists, but the foreign-born were not so very different. William Penn, Roger Williams, Tom Paine, Carl Schurz, were a few of those who, unable to make headway against all the débris and cynicism of the Old World, grasped the magnificent opportunities offered by this land for a better scheme of things.

The fame of attempts such as theirs re-echoed from our forest frontiers all the way back over the ocean, inspiring some of the unlikeliest people to hope of retrieving their fortunes, or enlarging their scope, or improving society, in this ample asylum of ours. Napoleon, after Waterloo, nourished fleeting intentions of playing the American provinces; Wordsworth and Southey dreamed up a state for poets to be founded on the banks of the Susquehanna. (Good poets that they were, they chose that site for the musical fall of its syllables.) Perhaps as many such dreams came true as failed of crossing the Atlantic.

The most grandiose little Utopia ever conceived in any sane noddle was actually transplanted here, to the banks of the Wabash, and took root long enough to give forth an unearthly blossom. New Harmony, in Indiana, was America's first and most ambitious experiment in total communism.

Every time I write of this place, I get a flood of letters beginning, 'Sir!' (and no 'dear' about it.) Half of these pen pals assume, before they have read past the word 'communism,' that I am advocating the overthrow of the United States Government, that I want the shiftless to get a share of my correspondent's savings, and that I must be living in sin with somebody. The other half, however, reading my same remarks, are wont to write me in this wise: 'I suppose you're one of those Fascists who would stab our Russian allies in the back. I am amazed at your ignorance. Don't you know that . . .' But the astonishing incident of New Harmony seems to me to prove nothing at all about communism, for or against.

And if my temperance about this social principle, and my disposition to see both good and evil in it, raises your blood-pressure, you might skip this chapter.

My interest in New Harmony, as one of the great little towns of America, was born when I learned that it was once the capital of the natural sciences in all the New World. When it had only a thousand souls in it, its streets were fuller of gifted naturalists than New York, Philadelphia, Boston, Washington. The Indian frontier was not a hundred miles off, in 1826, and the woods were still full of deer, when this startling center of enlightenment was producing scientific books that widened savants' eyes in Europe. It was said that so many eminent men had gone to New Harmony that the meetings of the Philadelphia Academy of Sciences became hardly worth attending. From this village set forth one of the first scientific exploring parties to cross the plains and reach the Rockies — a deed that has always sent my blood faster through my veins. In New Harmony, I had learned, was buried Thomas Say, one of my heroes of that expedition. He had come here as an eager young man, fallen in love and eloped with his Lucy, spent arduous years over his great life-work on the insects and birds and shells of America, received respectful visits from the scientific great of earth, and two princes beside, and finally admitted at his village door the last caller who comes to mortal man.

So New Harmony had been hallowed ground to me for years. It was for me one of those places that you find longingly on the map a hundred times; you wonder what it would be like really to walk in its streets, and look in the faces of its children, and breathe its remote air. Well, of course, it is easy enough to reach New Harmony or any other place in Indiana. But practically there are always a hundred prior claims on your time and your money; there is somewhere else that you must be, for one reason or another. So years may go by, the hope fade, revive, and fade again, before you actually see a signboard by the roadside, that says, in effect, that it's seventeen miles to your dream town. Or, in my case, *This Way to Little Utopia.*

From there on, every hill and tree reminds you that your great predecessors here also looked on this scene. And what was in their hearts, you wonder, that hurried their feet as they came by? Such reflections, if you are walking the Appian Way or climbing up to the Acropolis, may be appropriately answered by noble quotations. But what I sang, as I crossed the lush and placid Hoosier landscape, was a stanza from one of New Harmony's more glorious anthems:

> The day of peace begins to dawn.
> Huzza! Huzza! Huzza!
> Dark Error's might will soon be gone.
> Huzza! Huzza! Huzza!
> Poor mortals long have been astray,
> But knowledge now will lead the way.
> Huzza! Huzza! Huzza!

For the man who founded the town I was coming to started out with a declaration that 'the religious, moral, political, and commercial arrangements of society have been on a wrong basis since the commencement of history.' He proposed nothing less than to 'remodel the world entirely, and to root out all crime; to abolish punishment; to create similar views and similar wants and in this manner to abolish all dissension and warfare,' and thus remold this sorry scheme of things nearer to the heart's desire.

Moreover, he had the ways and means all worked out to a detail. One of the most telling blows toward clearing the ground of the imperfect society which now litters it was to be struck at the root of all evil; money was just to be done away with. This lofty reformer would issue a receipt for units of work performed, which could be exchanged at a non-profit, cooperative store. Every man would be taught to provide for his simpler necessities; trade, this Utopian planned, would then cease entirely. He purposed to do away with private property. Attributing prejudice and selfishness to the sentiments of the old-fashioned family, he proposed to take children from their parents at an early age and give them special training in service to the state.

Now the man who hatched out these projects was personally one of the gentlest, kindliest, most honest and generous of beings; the idea of violence in his revolution would have horrified him. It was the very character of their leader that strengthened the hopes of his followers. Born poor, in Wales, in 1771, Robert Owen had been himself a victim of the worst period of child slavery, and had fought his way up to wealth and power. In his model mill town at New Lanark, Scotland, he provided schools for employees still minors, and nurseries for the children of working mothers. He replaced slums with decent housing, and when his mills closed during a cotton shortage, he kept all hands on at full pay.

Yet in hard-headed Scotland his reforms were viewed with resentment. When he sought to arouse the public's conscience against child labor, he was accused of trying to weaken parental authority. Because he declared that women who married should retain legal rights in their own property, he was decried as coming between man and wife. When he told society that criminals are produced largely by criminal conditions (which Jane Addams was applauded for saying, a century later), those who did not want to face responsibility for the state of things cried out that he was chopping at the foundations of morality. His scheme for cooperative marketing and collective buying was viewed by business men as darkly dangerous. Because, though himself happily married, he suggested that the strict early-Victorian divorce laws might be eased, gossip had it that he advocated free love. So his name was slandered, and his hands were tied.

Owen turned to America. On that free and virgin soil, he believed, he could create a new kind of society. Before a tolerantly interested Congress, the Supreme Court, and President Monroe, he exhibited a model of his proposed town, and outlined the system he intended to set up there. Then, plunging his fortune into it and staking his reputation on it, he proceeded to put his theory into practice.

At 'Harmonie,' on thirty thousand acres along the Wabash, dwelt the Rappites, a sect of German peasants; they too were communists, of a religious order. Vowed to lives of celibacy, inured to back-breaking toil, thrifty, and skilled in handcraft, they had wrested their land from the wilderness, brought it into high cultivation, and here succeeded materially with their own monastic form of communal living. Guided with fatherly despotism by their shrewd and capable leader, Father George Rapp, they had become a self-reliant little society, producing almost all its own food, raising its own flax, cotton, and wool, out of which cloth was spun and woven and the people dressed. Their blacksmiths, masons, glass-makers, carpenters, millers, and other artisans provided every simple necessity and comfort. Tobacco and liquor they knew not; music and flower gardens were their only forms of self-indulgence.

It was a visit which Owen paid to these sober, industrious, highly skilled folk, contentedly awaiting the end of the world which, they were convinced, was at hand, that raised in the philanthropist such roseate hopes for his own brand of communism. So, for twenty thousand dollars, he purchased from the Rappites (who wished to remove to Pennsylvania) their orchards and vineyards and vegetable gardens, their fields of wheat and cotton and corn and flax, their fifty fine old houses, mills, granaries, factories, storehouses, and church, along with two hundred head of sheep, pigs, milch and beef cattle, and horses.

Thus magnificently equipped, and rechristened New Harmony, Owen's Kingdom-Come-in-the-Wilderness opened its doors and invited the world to enter.

And in no time at all the banks of the Wabash were fairly crumbling under the cheering crowds of those who still believed in Santa Claus. From all parts of the country they flocked, brought by every sort of motive. There were plenty of those who, though proven unfit to live in the world as it is, concluded that they would make ideal citizens of the world as it ought to be. Others were outright swindlers who played Owen for a sucker. There was also a solid backbone of honest idealists, some of them hard-working and willing to make great sacrifices for the good of humanity. Without these last the rest could scarcely have eaten, nor would they have felt impelled to stay over a week-end in what has been called the 'Town of Heart's Desire.'

To leaven this mass, there came at Owen's invitation a whole arkful of celebrated intellects, known to history as 'the Boatload of Knowledge.' Be it said at once that the only brilliant achievements made at New Harmony were those of its 'intellectuals,' who numbered among them some of the most gifted men and women of their times. Of these were Owen's sons. Robert Dale Owen was to become one of Indiana's most fearless and progressive legislators, a champion of the unrecognized rights of children and women. David Owen became an internationally famous geologist, whose mere presence in New Harmony was enough to move the headquarters of the United States Geological Survey thither, and to attract some of the most famous of Europe's scientists to his door. William Maclure, who as Owen's partner joined his fortune to the New Harmony enterprise, devoted his life to better education of the young and (half a century before Carnegie) to the establishment of free libraries. Frances Wright and Ernestine Rose were celebrated early feminists and abolitionists. Josiah Warren was the inventor of the rotary press on which all newspapers and magazines are printed today. And on board the ark *The Philanthropist* as it made its way through the ice that January in 1826, was not only Thomas Say, but Lesueur the ichthyologist and Gerard Troost the geologist. To such brave minds fell the tasks of school-teaching, lecturing, publishing the *Gazette*, and putting out the stream of magnificent scientific books which still make a volume with the New Harmony imprint a collector's prize.

But it was under a precarious and unprecedented social system that these fine minds had to function. The constitution which the New Harmonists now drew up is one of the curiosities of political history. It specifies that everybody is to have the same sort of food, clothing, and education, and all shall live in community houses. Anybody over twenty-one could participate in initiating and voting the laws, so that the whole citizenry constituted the legislative body, as in a small private club; no provision was made for electing legislators. Executive power resided in a council of elected delegates and officers; superintendents were appointed to different 'departments' — to wit: Agriculture, Manufactures and Mechanics, Domestic and General Economy, Literature and Science and Education. Property was to be owned in common. Everyone must labor, but instead of reward in proportion to worth, equal advantages were granted to all. New Harmony was to be conducted like one big happy family.

Only a week after I had stood where Boonesborough once stood, I found myself strolling the streets of a still extant New Harmony. They are leafy and stagnant streets; the town must sleep in dusty umbrage in the summer, but when I came in April the boughs were tenderly budded. The sweetness of an Ohio Valley spring day must have been the same as that a hundred-odd years ago, when the Owenites thought that a new morning had dawned for the poor old world.

Why this place should remind me of Boonesborough I couldn't think, as I explored it, unless it was because it was so different. But Transylvania and the Utopia of Robert Owen kept meeting in my mind. When with my finger I was trying to trace the obliterated inscription on Say's grave, it came to me that, just as engraving is the reverse of cameo, so the resemblance between these two towns of mine was a reverse one. Transylvania was the Kingdom Come of government by monopoly. New Harmony promised heaven on earth through communism. One was almost a mirror image of the other. For, though Henderson's basic belief was that it is every man's self-interest which holds the state together, and Robert Owen fondly proclaimed that society would be saved if everybody would gladly work for the other fellow's good, the effect of these two opposite philosophies upon their followers was much the same. In each projected scheme, the simpler souls all supposed that with the minimum of investment and labor, they would move right into easy circumstances for life.

Before we laugh at them too comfortably, remember that the Townsend plan still flourishes among many, and that others are fanatically convinced that the government is the enemy of their bank accounts. So it appears that Transylvania and New Harmony, too, are still with us; there is a little of both in my town and in yours.

Time, which has passed New Harmony lightly by, has neither destroyed nor materially cheapened it. Its population is about one thousand hospitable souls — almost what it was at the height of the Owenite glory and folly. Architecturally, the town is an anomaly in the state of the Raggedy Man, with its old Rappite buildings of three-foot-thick stone walls, hand-hewn beams, enclosed staircases, and Teutonic sturdiness lightened by the grace of long windows, simple columns, and honest proportions. With pride in the little that is left to them, and pleasure that someone has at last come to see it, descendants of the old families will show you the Owen-Maclure house, the Rapp community house, the frame dwelling where Say lived with his Lucy; they will point you out what was the tavern in Owen's time, and the opera house that has sunk to a garage. They will lead you with justifiable dignity past the gallery of dim likenesses salvaged from the years: Rapp's Old Testament, Kriss Kringle face, Maclure's countenance of the obstinate philanthropist, Owen's bigotty, kindly, Welsh phiz, ornithologist Say's brightly cocked eye and crown like a crested flycatcher's, and the loftily enlightened but opinionated features of Ernestine Rose and Frances Wright.

Utopia on the Wabash

But there was youth here, too, once upon a time, hopeful, perennial youth. Robert Dale Owen, in his delightful memoir, *Threading My Way*, tells what it was like for a young man in New Harmony when it was young.

> There was something especially taking, to me, at least, in the absolute freedom from all trammels, alike in the expression of opinion, in dress, and in social intercourse, which I found there. The evening gatherings, too, delighted me; the weekly meetings for the discussion of our principles, in which I took part at once; the weekly concert, with an excellent leader, Josiah Warren, and a performance of music, instrumental and vocal, much beyond what I had expected in the backwoods; last, but not least, the weekly ball, where I found crowds of young people, bright and genial, if not especially cultivated, and as passionately fond of dancing, as in those days, I myself was.

A young married woman, with more than her share of bodily drudgery in the New Moral World, has left us her record too. She writes a friend:

> I must inform you that our balls have never been put off for the most sultry night of the season. The young girls, too, here think as much of dress and beaux as in any place I was ever in.

The Duke of Saxe-Weimar, that inveterate visitor of curiosities, gives an aristocrat's view of innocent merriment unconfined:

> In the evening I paid visits to some ladies, and saw the philosophy of a life of equality put to a severe test with one of them. She is named Virginia (Dupalais), from Philadelphia; is very young and pretty; was delicately brought up, and appears to have taken refuge here on account of an unhappy attachment. While she was singing, and playing very well on the piano, she was told that the milking of the cows was her duty, and that they were waiting unmilked. Almost in tears, she betook herself to this servile employment, execrating the social system and its so-much-prized equality. After the cows were milked, in doing which the young girl was trod on by one and kicked by another, I joined an aquatic party with the

young ladies and some young philosophers in a very good boat upon the inundated meadows along the Wabash. The evening was beautiful, it was moonlight, and the air was very mild; the beautiful Miss Virginia forgot her stable experiences and regaled us with her sweet voice.

Now let us hear from a cynic, the anonymous-sounding Paul Brown:

> The dancing and the instrumental music engrossed more of energy than the important considerations of community welfare. There must be a regular ball and a regular concert once a week. The instituting of such amusements seemed to be propitious to interest the young and enamor them of the place. But the constant succession of this sort of thing clearly induced volatility and aversion to serious duties.

Further, the young woman earlier quoted began to lose her illusions:

> I for my part am pretty near out of my senses. It is impossible to express how completely miserable I am, nor how I can sufficiently deprecate my own folly in ever consenting to come so far at such an uncertainty.
>
> In the first place, all our elder children, those whom we expected to be comfort and consolation and support, in our old age, are to be taken away from us, at an age, too, when they peculiarly require the guardian care of their parents; and are to be placed in large boarding houses. The single males and females above the age of fourteen are to live together in one house, over which there is to be one married woman to superintend. Instead of our own dear children each housekeeper is to receive two more families, one of which will have a child under two years old. The rest will be at the boarding school. These three families are each to live in community, and take the cooking by turns. We have already got one family with us, but as the people are leaving the society very fast, I hope it will not be necessary to take a third. If it is, however, I shall prefer going into one of their miserable log cabins to being crowded too thick. I have hitherto been able to do very little besides sew and take care of my baby; and my health is now, as well

as my poor baby's, extremely delicate. How I am to go through cooking, washing and scrubbing I really do not know. But I know were I to consider this world only I would rather, far rather, that Mr. Owen would shoot me through the head.

The boarding schools into which the poor uprooted children were transplanted were conducted on the most progressive lines, one à la Pestalozzi, the other à la Froebel — (both of whom, it may be mentioned, received their first introduction into America via New Harmony). The scientifically moral hygiene of them starved the children for affection, and they were regimented past the endurance of young flesh. Some lived, under the watchful eye of a Mr. Neef, in the old Rappite community house, Number Two, which still stands; I climbed to the loft there where, so it was told me, the youngest once slept in little hanging cots and rejoiced nightly in the mischief of swinging the cots in unison so that they bumped one into another. Standing under the ancient timbers, I laughed aloud, for I remembered a wistful fragment those irrepressibles have left us — perhaps it was to this tune that they bumped their rebellious cradles:

> Number Two pigs shut up in a pen,
> When they get out, it's now and then,
> When they get out they sniff about,
> For fear old Neef should find them out!

'The children,' comments the scornful Mr. Brown, 'ran morally mad.'

On July 4, 1826, while Thomas Jefferson lay dying, the redoubtable Mr. Owen issued and read aloud in person a 'Declaration of Mental Independence,' to honor the fiftieth anniversary of the government he was so innocently trying to overthrow. Frances Wright was the speaker of the day. 'In Europe men have to fight for their independence,' she announced, but, she congratulated us, 'in America we have only to will it.'

The *New Harmony Gazette* outdid itself in rapturous report•

ing of her long speech. The *Gazette* indeed is a fascinating study in a controlled press on American soil. True, the editors were men and women of education, high intelligence, higher moral ambition; they never printed a scandalous story; they stooped to no yellow journalism or cheap effects of any sort; the contents of their sheet were meaty with ideas and unsullied with trivia and vulgarity. But they were writing sheer propaganda; they ignored all adverse weather signs; they refused to print opinions contrary to those which would advance their millennium. No mention of uncertainty, dissension, doubt, misery, unfairness, or maladjustment sullies their blue skies except for occasional references to the overcoming of past obstacles. Every week the clouds completely cleared up all over again, and the signals of fair weather were run up once more at the editorial masthead, as they had been the week before.

The secession of one group after another, who removed to other tracts in the neighborhood, is made to sound in the *Gazette* like the mushrooming of daughter colonies, all in accordance with Mr. Owen's sincere belief that the example of New Harmony would soon be imitated throughout the country, until the old selfish individual system of society was swiftly replanted by a selfless communistic one. Constitution after constitution was substituted at New Harmony, but the *Gazette* makes them seem merely like improvements amended upon the original document, instead of the desperate flounderings of a drowning idea.

For the millennium was showing alarming signs of departure. The moochers howled because, after all, they had to work. The industrious complained that as fast as the fruits of their toil accumulated, they were borne off by the parasitic. In a town which was supposed to have abolished money, people were ready to sell their souls for the feel of hard cash. New Harmony was a prohibition town, yet drunkenness was the commonest of sights in the streets, for stills operated on enclaves of private land.

When Father Rapp revisited the town, he must have shaken his head to see the fruit he had planted rotting on the ground because housewives were too busy pulling each other's hair to gather and preserve it. He found the weeds higher than the wheat and flax, the cattle recklessly slaughtered. The pigs had broken loose through unmended fences; they grubbed out the vegetables and dashed between the legs of a hundred amateur Platos arguing their pet republics in the streets. Where the Rappites had been a self-supporting community, with a surplus to sell to the outside world, the Owenites, unskilled or unwilling in agriculture and manufacture, had soon gone through their heritage, and before long they were compelled to buy clothing and food from the outside. They were unable to balance trade with any products except theories and talk.

All the irritation, confusion, waste, and misery in the Perfect State resulted in a popular demand that Owen should, 'until things got better,' accept practically dictatorial powers. But the only consequence was to make him personally, solely, and helplessly responsible for every real and fancied grievance, and for a thousand unpleasant or ridiculous failures which were the fault of everyone equally. Owen had pitted against him the operation of unrecognized economic laws which came into play as promptly as will the law of gravity when you step off a cliff. Yet there remains a residue of blame that Owen and his high-minded followers have to bear. For it has been said that total communism, to succeed, must rest on grace, as among the Rappites or the Shakers, or on force, as in Russia. Owen, a free thinker and a pacifist, took away the first and refused to substitute the latter.

So ordinary standards of moral responsibility in New Harmony deteriorated swiftly. The pursuit of happiness became a losing one. Bitterness grew. Where no one could develop inherent talents, since no provision or incentive existed for accomplishment, the only ambition of the New Harmonists was to survive — without hope of an improved status, and watching things go from bad to worse. Husbands got no more home cooking; enforced community living decreed that everyone must eat together in big dining halls, accepting what community kitchens turned out. (If it was a waste of brilliant young Robert Dale Owen's time to bake bread, it was a painful experience to eat his loaves.) Wives, ostensibly relieved of doing the family wash, might be drafted to work in the community laundry.

Bathos was reached when the leaders decreed a costume for all loyal New Harmonists — a sort of collarless smock for men, and baggy slacks for women, that set the simple pioneer neighbors of the community to guffawing. In fact, the whole country had begun to laugh, and this was the crackling, cleansing fire of American laughter which destroys all that is not proof against it.

At the sound of it, at the threatening sound of timbers giving way all through his fantastic edifice, Robert Owen did precisely what Richard Henderson did in Transylvania — he bowed himself out. Not without a magnificent exit speech, in which he assured his disciples of his hopes that, now he had shown them the plan for a perfect society, they would in his absence successfully execute it. Securely back in England, he assured audiences there, also, of the success of the New Harmony scheme; perhaps he reassured himself as well, for he returned to his Utopia in mingled hope and alarm. And now, even through such rose glasses as he wore, things looked utterly black. After all, he reproached his followers sorrowfully, the individualistic system had been too strong, his experiment premature. So, as promptly as possible, he left New Harmony forever, ruined in hope and fortunes; his fellow reformers too scattered like quail, to transfer their ideals to even more dubious experiments elsewhere.

The solid folk of New Harmony, after the dreamers and the moochers had gone, stuck with the town; they had come with hopes and they meant to realize something on them. So they were willing to make the difficult adjustment from an impossible economic system back to a stern one. This cost many of them a double price, just as Boonesborough's settlers had to start over again on fresh claims. It was men like David and Robert Dale Owen who stayed and faced the realities and shouldered the responsibilities. It was their kind who turned Utopia into Indiana, who woke out of a dream and looked on morning with eager eyes.

Robert Owen the dreamer was right, at least, when he proclaimed himself ahead of his time. We take for granted now much of what he tried to bring to us. Then we laughed at him for the fool he showed himself; we assumed, because his ship of state was glass, that all the cargo too must sink. Now we act as though we had invented the emancipation of woman, the protection of children from industrial exploitation, the abolition of slavery, public schools and compulsory education; we don't care to remember that a hundred years ago we opposed, from pulpit and newspaper, all these reforms proposed by Owen. Just when the need for them was greatest, we were hard-shelled about admitting that need. Our ancestors weren't especially to blame; it's always been that way, Heck, and if today you see somebody being stoned and cursed because he dares to tell us that we, the wise and good, must be better and wiser, you can get ready to tell your awed grandchildren that you knew that man 'when.'

That day I spoke at Rotary I saw your head lift nervously, Heck, when merely in passing I mentioned communism without the conventional curse on it. Since then Tovarish Stalin has dealt such thwacking blows on the back of Führer Hitler that a blessing on Russia has become almost as conventional. I can't make out whether the change of heart is sincere and lasting, or shallow and for the duration only. We thought we had Finland painted white and Russia painted red; now some hope that Russia may be more red, white, and blue than we'd supposed, and as for Finland, we have realized that it's not a forty-ninth state of the Union but just another one of those bedeviled European nations that make Uncle Sam pull worried at his goatee.

But, you know, we've found some communistic methods pretty useful in our own system. Your kids go to public school, don't they? Just as Owen hoped they would. Those schools are paid for by the community. In fact, even childless couples and people who send their children to private schools have to chip in tax money that's spent on the education of your children and your colored washlady's. The community also elects the school board; it goes farther: the truant officer can come right into your house, if you take a notion that you don't want your children to read and write, and fetch them back to the blackboard, and see that you're put in the jug to boot. Despotism, isn't it? And you don't notice much illiteracy around, do you?

Why, America's positively enthusiastic about some of its most communistic propositions! What would it say if the Department of Interior turned Yellowstone and the Grand Canyon back to private enterprise on a competitive basis? I fancy that the American people would march on Washington and pull the roof off the Capitol. Yet there are those — lumbermen, cattlemen, farmers, deer hunters, utilities promoters, and concessionaires — who hate the National Parks, who yowl that public ownership of these grand free areas is stifling business and spoiling sport. Nobody, however, pays any attention to their sorrows; every summer we come trooping back into the parks to have a good time.

The other day I saw, on the opposite side of my canyon, a farmer's chicken coop catch fire. To the tune of shrieking sirens the town's fire-fighting equipment with a highly trained and courageous crew dashed up the hillside to save incubator and pullets and roofing paper. Now, in the good old days before we got such communistic ideas in our heads, the proverbial Mr. Crassus made his pile by providing Rome with a fire brigade. If you smelled smoke, you sent for his outfit; the first to get to the fire was Crassus himself. He looked over your plant and he sized up your wad, and while the flames crackled he gave you an estimate of what it would cost to put them out. If you had the habit of haggling, or couldn't meet his price, he waved the bucket boys back to the station and let you burn down. Of course, a little free competition might have brought down the price, but it wouldn't have put out the fire in a poor man's house. Here in America even the people who live in fireproof houses with a sprinkler system installed have to pay taxes toward keeping the engines shiny. We don't mind admitting that our fire department is community-owned, and that it serves every man according to his need and not according to his ability to pay. But we do hate to hear the paint on it called red, even when it is.

That's because we hate the rash and barbarous suggestion that the national system we have built up must be torn down entirely in order to make room for the benefits that come with pooling things and working them out together. When anybody gets to talking that way too loudly around here, we rightly deport him. I'd like also to deport — to some vanished Transylvania where they'd have to begin from scratch with an axe — those paunchy individuals who are afraid to contemplate any improvements in our system for fear they might have to share in the bill for them.

Owen's New Harmony experiment, Heck, ought to settle your nerves about communism in America. Robust frontier health threw off the fever of it, yet kept what inspiration that fever gave. Maybe it does us good, once in a while, to get in a fever about things, to burn with anger at the rot still in us and thirst for our own betterment. We are a cool-headed people; even fevered for righteousness, I think, we shall commit no very great follies. We may achieve successes in brotherhood to astonish even ourselves, who have so far achieved so many. Let's not be afraid of a mere word, Heck. The important thing for you and me to see to is that America strides always in the vanguard of democracy. That will take hard, fast going. But Uncle Sam must never get a round belly.

14

Jim Bridger and the Bard

IF WE CAN LOOK COMmunism squarely in the eye, neither terrorized nor hypnotized by the red glare, it is because we are strong in what we are and have. But I remember how Russia looked to you, Baldur, when you came back from an eager visit to it. You had no homeland; behind you Germany had crumbled; France, for all her goodness to us, was only like a graceful week-end hostess, and we both knew it. But Russia had space and youth and hope, you thought, for the broken of Europe; you were on fire with the possibilities that you saw there for a new kind of life. 'It is so young, so big!' you told me, one of those evenings when we sat in the dusk under the yew tree by the Mediterranean. 'There is room there for a man to think. Nowhere can there be such wide, free room!'

You were too full of talk to care to listen, so I just pulled on my pipe and thought about Wyoming. Yes, and Montana, where the cloud shadows troop all day across the high plateaus and darken no doorstep. And Arizona, the miles and miles of hot sunny sand with not even a signpost. But I couldn't have explained; we were talking in French that night, I remember, because there was a pretty countess with us, and it doesn't sound the same when you call it '*le Far Ouest*.'

It's too big for mere description, anyway. Folks who live there don't care much about prettying it up with words.

When they talk, it's to tell you a yarn. About Sublette, maybe, or Broken-Hand Fitzpatrick, or Colter, who was the first man to see all hell broken loose in what tourists now call Yellowstone Park's geysers, though nobody would believe the tale when he got back to tell it. That was because the yarns in the West grow as tall as the men there. They're not fairy-tales, Baldur, like those of your Schwarzwald or the Lake of Annecy; the heroes we like best to yarn about really lived, and they were really heroes. Only, around the campfire, nobody minds if you stretch a point; everybody understands that to come near the true spirit you have to go high, wide, and handsome with mere fact.

So that's why I'd like to introduce you to the Far West by way of a yarn. I've stuck to the verifiable facts of each case all the way up to here, with here and there just a little filling in with color of the historical outlines. But now I'm hanging out a sign to say, about this chapter, Don't believe any more than you feel inclined. Not that it isn't most of it true, because all that's important to me in it is proven truth. But I did add an incident or two that isn't specifically in his biography, just to give you a better idea of what kind of a man Jim Bridger was.

Because he's my hero, and so tall of himself that I haven't added an inch to him, nor tidied him up; that Flathead squaw, for instance, is all Jim's. Already there are innumerable legends about him, and one more or less won't make much difference. Jim was large that way himself; as he once said, 'There ain't no bad whiskey in the world. All whiskey's good whiskey.' He had as liberal a thirst for stories; he longed for them, in the great loneliness of his life as hunter, trapper, and scout, in the days when everything west of the Missouri was Injun country. And Jim couldn't read. Now there's some real tragedy in that, and certainly the seed of a story. It sprouted in my mind when I discovered the uncontested fact that Jim somehow got hold of, and deeply prized, a set of Shakespeare. But he was dependent upon any 'eddicated' stranger who might pass to read it to him. I haven't a full transcription of Jim's critique of the Bard, but it is recorded that he opined that 'that there Fullstuff was too full of lager beer.'

You're a novelist, Baldur; you'll see that I couldn't leave such a hint alone. I'll let you know too, beforehand, that the other man in the story is a colored shadow cast by a true hero — but we'll come to that. The kid is my own youngest son with a red wig on. But there, you know how these tricks are worked; you do them yourself. They're the least of it; all that a writer constructs is merely the stone mouth through which an oracle may speak. We don't know where the voice comes from, but sometimes it comes blowing clear, and then you write down what it says. This time the story is borne on the wind, blowing from far away and years ago, sweeping between the Uintas and the Wind River Mountains of Wyoming, sighing emptily over the sagebrush. Then at last, in a pass where one lighted window shines, it finds the first and only outpost of humanity in all this empty West to talk to.

Around the angles of Jim Bridger's fort it lifted its lonely voice and, searching out chinks in the logs, it settled into a long soliloquy. It might have been speaking in blank verse or Comanche, for all a body could tell, but it sounded like someone with things to say to the man inside who was listening.

It would howl like an Indian boasting, then sink away soft as a whisper in a young girl's ear. What a lot of yarns it had to tell, if it would only tell them! All right, blow, blow, you old wind! Jim Bridger thought, angrily throwing buffalo chips on his fire. You and me been sassing each other a long time now. But I don't know your lingo, and all your huff and guff don't signify.

Here he was, settled down at last, at the forking of the Mormon Trail and the Oregon Trail. Here were lush grass and freckled shade under the aspens; there were trout in the stream, and even the birds sang as if this was just naturally a place for a dooryard and chimney, a place for a man to grow old in. So this was the spot he had chosen, when he saw the fur trade petering out, to set up his post by the side of the trail, his forge and his store and his rough log cabin. For the wagons were coming now, slow at first, like summer along the Green River, but just as certain, just as sure to be followed by harvest. Jim Bridger's trouble, queerly enough, was that this coming of people made him feel lonely, for the first time in his life.

He used to be friends with solitude. Trapping in the Bitter-roots and the Bighorns and the Tetons, he had loved it. A man wasn't lonely when he lay down at night with Danger for a wife, and hunted all day with Hunger for his squalling child. To go where no white man ever had been, to find the passes and open the mountains — that was the choice Jim Bridger made when he was no more than a boy. When he kissed the red-haired girl good-bye, and rode out of the town of St. Louis.

But now, after all, he had a home at last, and a woman in it. A Flathead squaw that talked Salish — when she talked; mostly she stared at him with her shoe-button eyes making heathen remarks he could no more savvy than the wind's. And when you had settled down, you wanted talk, you wanted yarning. You were hungry to hear about what had happened to other kinds of men, about old fights and elections and hangings, and all such doings. The folks going out to Oregon passed him gossip on their way, but it wasn't gossip that he wanted. He was looking again tonight at the book he had, and he saw that inside it must lie the stuff he hankered for. But Jim Bridger never learned to read or write.

This book, a thick volume in marbled binding, he had taken in payment for flour, off a woman whose husband died on the trail, because Jim was sorry for her. He was sorrier for himself, as he turned the pages in the firelight. For he couldn't find out what the pictures were about — this feller argifying at a skull, this nigger in a turban, this here drownded lady, and all the kings and queens. And that woman in her nightgown with a bloody knife in her hand — who'd she scalp? And why? To wonder was a tormentation. It ached in him like the Blackfoot arrowhead buried deep in his shoulder.

Jim Bridger, who could read sign sharp as any Indian, who held the whole chain of the Rockies printed in his brain, discovered that before this book he was a blind man. He could not walk here where other men went; he could not see what was plain to them; straining his ears for the stories in this volume, he heard nothing but the wind. He, who had so kindly a contempt for the tenderfeet passing in the wagon trains, was feeble as a baby before these pages. The weakness hadn't ever showed up as long as he kept going. The merchants in St. Louis, when he trekked back to lay in his stock, never thought of laughing when so famous a hero out of the Rockies could not sign his name or read a bill of sale. But tonight, poring ignorant over his book, Jim Bridger felt like a wolf looking through a window at a family within — a wolf that would like to get inside and become no better than a dog. He sees in that inner brightness the people moving, he knows they talk, but he can't understand, and they don't let him in.

Jim slammed the covers together, wishing he'd never taken the thing into his life to plague him. The thud caused the Flathead woman to look over her shoulder at him, where she stood at the window. He got from her one of her ungodly glances, and then she slowly turned her head with its square fall of coarse black hair back to the window and continued to gaze out fixedly. Interest was so rare in her that Bridger got up from the warmth of the fire, wondering what there could be to look at, out there in the black wastes.

Mrs. Cow-in-the-Sky Bridger, known to her husband in moments of rare tenderness as 'Peanuts,' may well have had her loneliness too, her own hankerings. Whether the people who came to her door were red or white, she was not at ease, being now neither one thing nor another, so she hid this under stolidity. Jim had to thrust her aside from the tiny square of glass which was their parlor window.

There in the east hung the morning star, and there below it leaped a glow now whipped high by the wind, now sinking between buffets. It shone damnation red, and it burned where there was no timber to catch, no rooftree, only a track in the sage where the wagon trains came bringing settlers.

Jim turned on Cow-in-the-Sky. 'Why in 'tarnation didn't you holler? That's folks in trouble, on the North Platte trail!'

She folded her arms impassively over her solid breast, as she watched him snatch his boots up from the hearth and jam them on.

'What's more,' he scolded, stamping into a heel, 'that's Injun work, and you know it.' He slammed on his hat and seized his gun. 'Sometimes I think I married a rattlesnake.' The door banged after him, and the night wind swept along with him as he raced for the corral.

It whistled him on as he covered the miles of dark and desert. The faster he rode, the smaller grew the blaze, for the fire was eating its feast up. It was only an evil glow in the sage when he came near enough to begin circling; the bravest man in the Rockies was no Indian's fool, to ride into the light of a burning wagon train, a mark for a Sioux arrow. But the night was dying, like the fire; the stars were gone; the spawn of darkness might have got themselves off by now, with their bloody trophies dangling at their hard thighs. Pacing his mare to a cautious walk, Jim made the circuit of the fire; he sniffed as he went, at the hateful smell of leather and cloth in cinders, and of singeing ox flesh; he peered when the wind picked up the last of the flames and lit the bodies. They lay flung about, in their decent skirts, their honest boots, with the pitiful look of life still on them. Nothing stirred but the sage in the rising dawn wind. One more of the smouldering wheels cast its iron rim; the embers crackled and spat their last; the dark was fading, and Jim swung down from his saddle. He stood in the midst of the dead with his hat in his hand, looking east where they had come from, where the light was coming.

Yes, the day, a summer day eerie with sweetness, was stealing over this charnel horror. Soon the old sun would come up, all good-natured and telling you what a fine morning it was; already the meadowlarks were hollering one to another, gay as a passel of schoolgirls. Jim Bridger, who had seen his fill of violence and done his share of killing, was sick with the dirty fury of this attack, and hot in his heart with defiance.

'I opened up this here pass,' he said aloud, 'for the folks to come through. And there ain't nothing, this side o' hell or the other, is going to keep 'em back.'

He spoke to wilderness and the dead and the retreated red men waiting again to murder. But there beyond that clump of sage, the lid of a toppled trunk began to lift. Out of it peeped a topknot colored like the sunrise, and then two eyes, dollar-big in their sooty sockets that stared at Jim Bridger, blue as the brightening sky but still filled with black horror.

Jim's startled smile broadened to a grin, and he stepped as gingerly as to a little bird that might fly from him. 'Open it up, son,' he said gently. 'Come on out. It's all safe now. They've gone, and it's just Jim Bridger.'

Throwing off the blankets that had buried him, a skinny little boy emerged from the trunk with spider agility. He looked around him wildly once, then flung up the crook of his arm to hide from himself what he saw, his small body shaking as if a violent gust blew through it. Jim caught him up and swung the two of them into the saddle. 'Get on, Chinook girl,' he said in the mare's ear. 'Get me this blessed brat out o' the hell they made him!' And the earth of Wyoming thudded in spurts of dust under the flying hoofs.

'Angus McClaren McClaine' was a heap of name for a tad, so Bridger called him 'Firetop.' 'It'll be easier for me to remember,' he said. He didn't tell the child that that was the name he'd had for the last white girl he ever kissed.

Firetop neither assented nor objected. It seemed at first that he couldn't get the breath in his throat to talk with. The youngster was scared stiff, for a fact. You would have said he'd died with the others, but for the enormous shine of his eyes. They followed Jim all around the room. And when Jim went out, he'd find on getting back that Firetop and Peanuts were backed into opposite corners, watching each other like a fox cub and a coyote. One scared and the other jealous, thought Jim, and he clapped his wife around her sullen shoulders, and hoisted the boy to his own.

Jim kept waiting for the kid to sob it all out, and tell how it had happened and who the folks had been. But the boy didn't let a word about the massacre pass his set sharp little teeth, nor a tear fall from those scorched blue eyes. Guts to that kid, Jim admired. He asked the boy's age, and the child said, 'Nine,' and, asked where he came from, said, 'York State. Cattaraugus County.' The thoughts that went on behind those big harebell-blue eyes Bridger could no more read than the print of his book.

Jim Bridger didn't hurry a body. The less a man talks, he knew, the more you can rely on what he says. And time wasn't much more to Bridger than to an Indian. Still, it was his plain duty, he supposed, to get the boy back to what might be left of his family, somehow. But, pressed, Angus Firetop explained that his ancestors were in Scotland; there didn't seem to be a soul this side of the Atlantic he belonged to.

Well, then, thought Jim, I don't have to keep nudging the Lord for an eastbound wagon. And that's a good thing, for they don't come often. 'So it was out to Oregon you was bound, bub?' he queried, dropping his trout line carefully into the Black Fork. 'There's a lot of good folks going that way. Do you want I should fix it up for you to go on with some of 'em?'

The boy, sitting with his fish pole in his two scrawny hands, staring in the water at things that weren't in it, said, 'No.'

A band of happiness devils jumped out of the alders and gave old Jim's heart a turn. He watched them twinkle away on the brooklet's riffles, and such a light spread on his own face in a slow grin of realization.

Firetop suddenly grabbed his pole as it slithered through his hands; the trout, describing an arc like a rainbow's, flipped with a wriggle into his eager grasp. Jim yelled hooray, and the fox-cub face turned up to him brimming with sudden light. Why, the kid looked happy! And all the June day blurred and shimmered between Jim Bridger's blinking lids.

For the boy had hooked him as neatly as he hooked that trout. He tagged along so close Jim got to feeling he was part of himself. They did together the things Jim always had done, in the forge and the store and the corral. All his life Jim Bridger kept his own hours; he ate when he was hungry, he slept when he was tired, and he got up again when he'd slept himself out, like a bear that shakes his hide and blinks without astonishment at the morning star.

There never was a boy in the world who wasn't sick of washing his hands for dinner and going to bed at bedtime. So Firetop seemed to think Jim's was the finest way in the world to live. The newness of it perked him up considerably. He even began to eat a bit, and Jim took a fatherly pride in that. He would put more flesh on that youngster's bones than they'd done back in Cattaraugus County!

Their silence seemed companionably good to the man of the wilderness. He did not see that the child was holding himself in, being too brave for his age. A woman might have known how to break that terrible courage to let healing in, but Cow-in-the-Sky belonged to a race to which stoicism was natural. So she shoved the boy a platter of jerk and meal, and said nothing.

'Ever been to school, Firetop?' asked Jim, by the way, when they had finished their midafternoon breakfast.

Angus nodded.

Jim looked at him, took his pipe out of his lips, and cocked his head as a wonderful inkling dawned. 'Couldn't be you could read, could it?'

''Course,' said the small boy briefly.

Jim heaved up and strode to the shelf where the book

Jim Bridger and the Bard

leaned on the whiskey bottle. The fat volume parted at the well-thumbed picture of the lady dripping blood from her knife. Jim laid it open on the child's sharp knees, thumping the print with a big forefinger. 'Read it,' he commanded. 'Read me all it says about that there!'

Firetop bent to the page, and piped up clear and fluent:

> 'Out, damned spot! out, I say! — one; two; why, then 'tis time to do 't. — Hell is murky!'

Jim started in a double amazement. Hell and damnation, was it? And was reading so easy?

> 'Yet who would have thought the old man to have had so much blood in him?'

'Go back,' Jim ordered, jabbing the page feverishly. 'Go back to the beginning. Let's have the whole murder, lynching and all.'

Witches, supernatural storms, ghosts, owl-haunted castles — he heard of them all through words like a rising wind. Clashing swords, lordly banquets, marching armies, and a knife in your back while you slept. Sleepwalking, and blood that wouldn't wash out. Trees that could travel, and vengeful thanes.

'What's a thane, do you reckon?' asked Jim with his hands on his knees and his eyes wide as Firetop's.

Angus McClaren McClaine knew that one.

'I see,' nodded Jim. 'A big chief, in your folks' country. Well, get on with the yarn. I don't get half the lingo, but it beats an Ogallala chief for laying it on grand and solemn.'

The sunlight went; the twilight came; the boy took the book to the window. The dark fell; he read on obediently by fireshine. At last Jim Bridger heaved the sigh of a man full-fed after famine. 'I never did hold,' he ruminatively commented, 'with letting a woman handle weepons.'

Now began an orgy, a madness, the most continuous season of Shakespeare ever produced. Firetop read himself hoarse, happy in service to his god; whether he understood the lines himself or not, he gave them all that eloquence natural to the highly imaginative. Jim smoked and drank and listened, and filled his pipe again, and bade the boy go on. Then at the end he would tumble the child with him into his buffalo robes, be it night or morning, reeling with the fumes of the most glorious language ever written, and somewhat, also, with the corn liquor he'd taken 'to clear his head,' as he claimed.

Cow-in-the-Sky in her corner stared opaquely; she fed them and otherwise kept out of their way, for she could hear in the little boy's eerie voice that he was talking with spirits:

> 'Angels and ministers of grace, defend us!
> Be thou a spirit of health or goblin damn'd,
> Bring with thee airs from heaven or blasts from hell,
> Be thy intents wicked or charitable,
> Thou com'st in such a questionable shape
> That I will speak to thee —'

Outside in the night a wind that had lifted its voice around the coigns and castellations of Elsinore besieged Jim Bridger's cabin with a moan like a kingly ghost's. The stars brightened and the stars paled over Wyoming, and the mightily marching verses strode over the sky with them and bade them vanish at the end of the play. Jim lay back on his buffalo hides, the bottle empty in his hand, in his head a fullness of fate and philosophy that left him almost sober as dawn came tiptoeing through the pass.

The fox cub lay curled at his hero's feet. He was trembling, sleep retreating in a relentless ebb from his exhausted brain. Not for nothing was the boy a Celt. Death, destiny, honor, madness, genius, they were so many winds that smote the strings of his heart. Inside his child's imagination, that had been blooded by a terrible reality, the drama projected itself long after the Bard (penning the perfect ending and knowing it with an artist's satisfaction) had intended the murky business to stop. The rest was not silence in the little red head, but Jim Bridger snored right through it with an innocence greater, for all the nicks in his gun, than this odd and brilliant child's.

Sometimes it did cross Bridger's mind that the boy might be missing a mother. But shucks, he thought, Peanuts is good to him. He's got around her. As for himself, his heart was soft and big within him toward the boy. He sat looking at the morning light on that bent bright crest, thinking it was the color of hair he'd have chosen for a son of his own. The little reed of a voice piped on:

> 'All the world's a stage,
> And all the men and women merely players.
> They have their exits and their entrances;
> And one man in his time plays many parts —'

Now it appears I'm father to this boy, thought Bridger happily.

> '— creeping like snail
> Unwillingly to school —'

Hell, he's got book-learning enough already, Jim agreed. 'Reputation at the cannon's mouth,' eh? I'll teach him how to use shooting irons. There's plenty Indians on up the Big Horn need shooting. A wise judge, did the book say? Well, the kid might get to be a judge, at that; he's smart enough. The gorgeous passage rolled to an end, and Jim nodded. When it was played out, 'this strange eventful history,' you could go peaceful if you'd raised a boy to take your place.

Jim Bridger, the wariest scout in all the West, forgot to listen for approaching danger. For now the lover climbed to the balcony of his sworn enemy's daughter. Now the fairies stamped, quarreling, in the moonlit dew. Now a king offered all he owned for a fresh mount, and couldn't get one nowheres. The Jew sharpened his knife on his sole; the Roman fell in his own blood; the old king tottered weeping through the sagebrush, and the ruined autocrat in the red robes bade the cabin walls

> 'Farewell, a long farewell, to all my greatness!'

'Hesh up, bub!' broke in Jim Bridger, turning a keen ear to the wide outside. 'That's wheels comin' up from the Platte.'

The emigrant train camped out a night in the little green valley, and Jim was visited that evening by some of the folks, a Reverend Whittemore and his wife, that Firetop had made friends with. Nice folks as you'd ever want to see; Bridger warmed to them himself. The other wagons went on next day, but the Whittemores said they must wait over for the next train rolling west, for one of their oxen was too badly galled to haul the Conestoga. So Bridger made them welcome to the empty storeroom in the cabin, and to his table.

At first he really believed it was that ox that delayed them. He was glad to have them; it all made good business for him, and the Reverend Luke Whittemore struck him as a cuss all of a man's size even if he was pious.

'Talk about brave, Reverend! A customer like you has got more gall'n I have — stoppin' to pray over an Injun when you could sooner shoot him!'

Deep in the long black beard a smile warmed the stern lips. 'We are all children of the Lord, even the savages.'

Jim, who knew Indians, was sure the Devil had fathered them, but there was a kind of Old Testament grandeur about the Reverend that, like the lingo of Shakespeare, convinced you of what you knew couldn't be true. If he had respect for the tall gaunt preacher, he felt a qualm that was near to timidity before Martha Whittemore. The very rustle of her starched skirts around this cabin made a pigsty of it, and yet she was all kindness, all decency and good manners.

'Mrs. Bridger,' she would say to Peanuts in the politest, neatest manner of speaking, 'if I might have a little more of your excellent meal mush? You must show me how you prepare it so tastily.'

And Jim, who knew Peanuts too, and the sort of black and bloody thoughts moving behind her lava-blank eyes, had the feeling at the back of his neck you get when you're ambushed. Because Firetop took to the Whittemores all too natural.

He cursed himself for having been so confidential with them about the boy, right off, the first night setting round the fire. 'Never hev heard a whimper out of him about the whole thing yet,' he had concluded proudly. 'Close-mouthed as an Injun, that boy.'

The terrifying look of a good woman bound to do good to somebody had leaped up in Martha Whittemore's eyes. But she spoke as smooth as a gopher snake slipping into its hole when she answered placidly:

'Well, Mr. Bridger, you've done your part, I'm sure. That's a smart boy, and deserves a good Christian raising.'

That night when the Reverend read from the Bible and then prayed aloud for God to prosper His word among the heathen, Jim prayed silently for the good Lord to send another westbound wagon train quick.

But Divine Providence was slow to act, and one day followed another at little Fort Bridger. Mrs. Whittemore took the opportunity to do a large washing, in the Black Fork; a smell of soap mingled with sage on the wind, and a long line of bright clean clothes flapped signals to any Sioux watching from the hills. Bridger, in the corral, could see Firetop sitting on an upturned bucket by the brook, talking with the missionary's wife as she pinned up shirts and petticoats. Jim whistled, but the boy didn't seem to harken. Chinook got a short-tempered slap on her rump and galloped off with a feminine toss of her head. Yet Bridger couldn't rightly say the Whittemores were trying to get at the child any. They minded their own business, but it had a powerful attraction for the youngster.

It didn't make things a bit easier under Jim's skin that in these last days that Blackfoot arrowhead in his shoulder got to tweaking and twisting like the Devil's pincers. The prophetic eyes of the Reverend Whittemore were fixed more often on Bridger when he writhed of a sudden under internal torment. It seemed sometimes that man could look right under Jim's shirt and hide, even into his conscience. A cuss word broke from Jim in spite of himself.

'Sorry, Reverend,' he said hastily, 'I've got a bit of Injun deviltry left stuck in my shoulder from a ruckus couple years back. Seems when the wind blows the wrong way it kinda bites me.'

'Our devils must be cast out,' replied Whittemore with a grave sympathy. 'Perhaps you will let me help you?'

Jim reached a rueful hand around and caressed the spot that hurt him. 'Thank you kindly, Reverend, but I guess it's jest something I got to bear, and I don't know but what I'd miss it ef it was gone.' He spoke with a certain defiance.

And yet when he got the boy off by himself one day, in the sage and the wind and the vast candid sunshine, Jim Bridger's conscience prodded him to speak up honestly at last.

'Firetop,' he blurted to the child in the saddle before him, 'how'd you like to take up with the preacher and his wife, 'stead o' me?'

Over his shoulder the boy flung him one look. It searched Jim Bridger's sorrowful eyes to the bottom. Then he turned from the pommel and flung his arms around the stony-faced plainsman.

'I won't ever leave you!' he passionately promised. 'Not ever.'

So Jim rode back at a gallop, and pulled up Chinook on her hinders with a flourish before his door. Well, now, he guessed it didn't matter how long they stayed, and he came in to supper, Firetop on his shoulder, in a mood of defiant good will. He had to eat regular these days, and put up with a grace too, but he was tolerant now, confident; his pride went before him, cardinal-red.

The fall was not Jim's, but Firetop's. He rose from the hearth where he stumbled, blood dripping from the gash in his brow that the hook of the crane had made there, and Bridger cried out heartily,

'Well, now, ain't you a sojer! Not a tear out of you! Skin ye alive, and you wouldn't whimper, would ye?'

Up rustled Martha Whittemore briskly. 'We'll just put a

bit of rag and some arnica on it.' She bent to the boy with such tenderness in her good face that the child's lips quivered and a great sob broke from him like a flood through a broken dyke.

'Here, here!' cried Bridger, shaken, but the woman took the little boy up in her arms and carried him, loudly weeping, out, closing the door behind her.

Jim turned, as in the next room the tempest rose, and met the merciless and pitying eyes of the missionary. They confronted each other in silence; from beyond the closed door a passionate treble struggled through sobs, and both men stood rooted, at the words. For now the whole terrible story of the attack before dawn in the sagebrush came pouring out hysterically, broken only by pauses when the child reached to the bottom of his lungs for another life-giving breath, till at last the horror died away, spent in the child's steady weeping for his mother.

'It's a mighty shame this had to happen,' said Jim lamely. 'I wouldn't have thought a bump and a scratch like that would have broke him down and brung it all back.'

'At last he could cast out his devils, poor babe,' answered Whittemore gently. 'They have been torturing him — haven't you seen it, man? You're a famous hero, James Bridger, for your own great courage. But a child can bear just so much.'

Jim looked around him desperately for a way out of this; his eyes found the whiskey bottle, and slunk back to the gaze of the bearded prophet. 'Nobody knows much about children when he's fust a father,' he said defiantly. 'Reverend, that boy's like a son to me.'

'But you have no mother to give him,' replied the missionary.

Bridger looked down at his boots for a moment. For himself, he would never be ashamed of Peanuts. The Great Salt Lake's desolation, the ice of the Medicine Bows, the bubbling hells at the source of the Yellowstone — he could never have asked the red-haired girl to share that. So he lifted his eyes boldly and said,

'The boy hisself says he wants to stay with me.'

Whittemore smiled. 'He's properly grateful.'

'You think he don't mean it?' Jim's anger rose, because he was beginning to be frightened.

'Perhaps he does,' said the preacher judicially. 'But a child cannot decide, Mr. Bridger, what is best for him.'

'I can tell you what's good for him,' Bridger declared. 'A fine healthy body, a life that makes a man brave enough to face hell if he must, a trigger finger and an eye for sign. That's what's opened the passes. I'll make the boy the best scout on the plains.'

'You are that yourself, sir, and the whole nation is bounden to you for it.' Whittemore gripped the chairback as if it were a pulpit and would give him a power he needed. 'But our children, Mr. Bridger, have a different task than ours. They will grow up in the best world we can make for them, but it is their duty to their country and their God to make it a better one, and far different, than this savage-ridden waste.' He flung the chair from him, and strode to the other man, clapping him on the shoulder with an earnest simplicity. 'Give us the boy, Bridger, I beg it of you! Not because my wife's a childless woman — not to comfort our sore hearts for that. But because he's a lad with a brain and a soul in a thousand. He'll be a man, if he's taught, to lead our people into the New Canaan and make straight a path in the wilderness.'

Whittemore's eyes were shining with a selfless fire. Jim stared into them, his own pupils drawn down to a bead inimically. The preacher dropped to his knees and his voice rose over the subsiding snuffles in the next room. 'O Lord, let Thy light shine upon this man in his darkness and open his eyes to Thy wisdom!'

'By God,' cried Jim in wrath, 'I won't be prayed over. Get up and let's settle this like men, Reverend!'

Whittemore sprang to his feet. 'Don't you blaspheme, James Bridger! The Lord is watching us. You're afraid of Him, that's what!'

Jim lifted his arm — to do, he was never to find out quite what. For a sudden pain, more terrible than any he had ever known, shot through that shoulder, and Jim's curse streaked blue across the air. You could smell brimstone for a second.

'My poor fellow!' said Whittemore after a moment, softly. 'You must have that arrowhead out. Come, trust me.'

Jim set his teeth and shook his head. 'I'll keep my arrowhead, thank 'e.'

'And what for?' pursued the man of God relentlessly. 'Is James Bridger telling me he's afraid to have it out?'

Their eyes met again, and Bridger saw it was true — it was God he'd been scared of. God shining in those eyes, showing Jim his way like a lantern. He spoke in a voice grown steady and sweet. 'I'd be mighty obleeged to you, sir, if you'll use the knife on me.'

Jim Bridger got through it by holding fast to the thought of how hard it must be for the Reverend to do. Only a man who trusted in the Lord could have got out that iron with the cartilage grown over it. Whittemore soundlessly prayed as he worked, and because there was silence in the next room, never a groan escaped the Blackfeet's victim. In her habitual silence Cow-in-the-Sky held the basin, brought the medicine man the iron she had heated at his order, and looked on as the wound was cauterized against gangrene.

So that Angus Firetop, gone blessedly to sleep against Martha's bosom, did not know what had been done between the two men. He was rolled into bed with his clothes on, while the sun was still high, and he slept right through the night till next sun-up. He did not hear the wheels of the westbound wagons that rumbled to a halt before Bridger's fort, or the sound of the camp made in the alders. But in the morning, waking from the long, purifying sleep that effaces nightmare, Angus found that he was being washed, for the first time in weeks, and combed and mended by Martha Whittemore. There was a happy stir in the air, and he was a part of it, for, without knowing how he had decided it, he found that he'd said, yes, he wanted to go on to Oregon. With his hand so warmly held by Mrs. Whittemore, Angus knew he spoke the truth.

Standing in his cabin doorway, watching the white-topped wagons roll away to the west in their golden dust, Jim Bridger said to himself, Well, anyhow, he cried when he left me. The smile he had made so hearty for Firetop at the last lay faintly still on his lips. Some day, some way, he thought, that tyke'll be a big man in the Oregon country. A wagon topping the rise suddenly showed a distant flutter of white, a handkerchief waved high with a gay and adventurous flourish. Jim lifted his hand in an answering signal.

> 'Forever, and forever, farewell, Cassius!
> If we do meet again, why, we shall smile;
> If not, why then this parting was well made.'

Bridger could not remember just how any of the words went, but there rolled through his head the surge of a noble sorrow. He turned and entered his cabin, and went to the shelf to find solace. But it was not the whiskey he got down; it was the book, and in his hands it opened to that picture of the sad man handing over his crown to some other fellow. Jim pondered the print, with a sheepish hope that, now he'd heard it read once, somehow it might come clear to him. But it was all just crow tracks. Yet suddenly he could hear the voice of Firetop piping up, about in here:

> 'For God's sake, let us sit upon the ground
> And tell sad stories of the deaths of kings.'

Jim shut the book abruptly. 'For God's sake, let's not!' he said aloud with vigor. He stood holding the volume in his two hands, reverent of it, but done with it. They were great yarns, and he was proud to have heard them. But all that happened long ago, if it did happen; it looked to him now, when he thought of what Firetop might live to see, little and far away, bright-colored and rubbishy. We've got no kings here, I'd like to tell the feller wrote this, Jim thought, gripping the volume as if to communicate with it; we're all free men. This here's America. An enormous, inarticulate eloquence swelled in him. He lifted his scout's eyes to the long, bellying sweep of the clouds across the horizon, out there beyond his little window. Why, what I've seen and done is just a beginning to the grandest story of them all! That farsighted gaze narrowed and filled with light. Jim Bridger stood staring at his country's future — print that he could not read, poetry greater than Shakespeare's.

15

Marcus and Narcissa Whitman

THE STATE OF WYOMING is a saddle, a big western saddle thrown over the backbone of the continent. The lowest spot is over three thousand feet high, and the peak of the pommel is more than thirteen thousand feet into the clean air. Out in Wyoming is where we brew our blizzards; those storms made of hard pellets of old snow gouged out of the ten-foot drifts, mingled with soft blinding new snow, hurtle along in subzero temperatures on a sixty-mile gale that may kill any living thing exposed for more than a couple of hours to its full fury.

And out in Wyoming is where Nature nourished the fiercest Indians in all our story of Indian fighting, that is written over three hundred years, on a page three thousand miles broad. That's where the Ogallala Sioux and the Teton Sioux danced for war and buffalo and rain; that's where the relentless Comanches and the roaming Cheyennes and the deadly Arapahoes lived, and the gentlemanly Crows. All the western tribes lived up to that idea of the redskins which is now so full of delicious terror; they wore war bonnets of eagle feathers, and they lived in tepees of buffalo hide. They rode like arrows from the bow, and they circled and they whooped before they closed in on you.

The long ranges of Wyoming plow north and south, always with those vast hollows of light air between them.

You can see them from so far away that you feel as though you were sighting mountains on some other planet and are amazed that there too, so far out in space, there are forests of pine and spruce, and snows with unimaginable little flowers at their feet. When the chinooks — the thaw winds — blow, coaxing those flowers up, they whisper the names of Wyoming's mountains: the Big Horns, the Medicine Bows, the Laramies, the Absarokas, the Wind Rivers, the Grand Tetons. And they sigh to remember great chiefs who were kings here, Sitting Bull and Red Cloud and Washakie.

Now, for all its snows and all its painted warriors, Wyoming lay across the path of American destiny. Southward, in Colorado, there were mountains even more impassable; farther south, in New Mexico, was the power of Spain, with an old antagonism and a deadly fear of the American advance. Northward there was Montana, with its passes locked in ice except for a few months in the year, and beyond that lay Canada, where the Hudson's Bay Company, polite as it was firm, was determined to keep the Yankees from reaching Oregon.

And Oregon, by which men then meant the state of Washington too, had become in our minds that earthly heaven to which good Americans might go before they died — if they didn't die on the way. It was the green mirage that would stand still and let you come to it, and rise up solid, when you got there, in giant groves of fir and cedar, hemlock and sugar pine. It would be water after Wyoming's thirst; it would be black soil after the alkali and loess. Not prickly pear, but ferns; not buffalo, but a place for the herds to come lowing back to full barns.

First, explorers saw it, Lewis and Clark and Captain Cook, Vancouver and the American whaling captains who came all the way around the Horn. After the explorers, in American history, you'll always find the trappers coming, men like Jedediah Smith, and old Joe Meek — Kit Carson's side-kick — Carson himself, of course, and Charbonneau who had been Sacajawea's papoose, and Hugh Glass that was killed by a bear and came to life to hunt down the men who deserted his mangled body. And you wouldn't want to forget old Bill Wolfskill who laid out the California Trail, or Vandenburgh, king of the fur trade, whom the Blackfeet rubbed out, or Tom Jackson who found Jackson's Hole — a 'hole' is a great valley between peaks — or Pete Ogden, the Hudson's Bay man that found Ogden's Hole. Then there's Pierre the Frenchman, and Bent of Bent's Station, his fort piled to the roof with beaver and martin pelts, and Broken-Hand Fitzpatrick — why, stranger, I couldn't be telling you about all these old-timers; the yarns are too long.

After the trappers it's always the missionaries. But there is always a quarrel between those who want to save the souls of the natives and those who want to exploit them. This explains the rotten eggs hurled by the Missouri River trappers at Doctor Marcus Whitman when he traveled westward in 1834 toward Wyoming on his way to Oregon. This Whitman, however, was less a theologian than a medical missionary; indeed, he was the man who really cut the arrowhead out of Jim Bridger's back. Perhaps I took his name a little too lightly in my last chapter, giving it a twist, but the incident happened, for a fact. It happened in the summer when the trappers and traders of all the West held their annual rendezvous on the banks of the Green River in southwestern Wyoming. That was the summer when Kit Carson came to the rendezvous and saw Singing Grass the Arapaho girl. And it appeared in that year that there were a lot of flints and lance points left in men's backs; yes, and there was cholera on the plains that summer. It's bad enough when a death like that comes to a thickly populated country, stalks into hospitals and crowds the morgues; it's even more uncanny when it drifts invisibly through places wild and clean and open, when men have to writhe and die alone under the stars or sun.

To those traders and trappers, the hardiest men on earth —

the Mountain Men, as they called themselves — the thirty-two-year-old Doctor Whitman, who had studied theology as well as medicine, looked like a healer sent by God. By God, sir, he was a man after all. He made you down your dose as relentlessly as your ma did when you were a kid; and if this was to be your last ride, he seemed to know where the trail was heading. Just where the Mountain Men were tough, this fellow was gentle as a girl back home; just where they were easygoing and careless, he was exact and stern with them. How did they like that? Well, they came back for more, didn't they? So he was 'big medicine' at the rendezvous, at Council Bluffs, and in the old South Pass. When he went back East to rouse the Protestant missions to their call among white men and red in the West, he left behind him friends among the Mountain Men who would guide him anywhere, furnish him whatever he needed, or promise to meet him any moon he'd name, on any sandbar in the braided Platte, or coulee in all that western nowhere.

Far across our heathen land, upon the pious Ararat of Cornhill, Boston, resided the American Board of Control for Foreign Missions, hereinafter to be known as the Board. Its Secretary was the Reverend Doctor David Greene, a cultivated man, a courteous gentleman; in the likeness I have of him here he seems sweetly conscious of the light of blessing bestowed by the photographer or God on his domed bald brow. To the Board Doctor Whitman made application for the opportunity to found a new mission in Oregon. They say that the Board was upset by Whitman from the beginning; returned home from that first western trip, on a Sunday morning, he had marched down the church aisle with two fierce-looking Nez Percé boys heeling him. Now, most of the good souls who supported the Foreign Missions by their contributions regarded the American Indians as vermin. If they ever thought of the Mountain Men, it was as damned past saving. They greatly preferred that their dollars should buy hymn books for Zulus, since the Zulus might remain a comfortably abstract means to grace. Unfortunately, however, the Zulus that year had gone to war, and were not interested in hymn books. And the story was going around the country that a delegation of Flathead Indians from Montana had come all the way to St. Louis to ask the white fathers to send wise men to their people, bringing the Word of God.

After waiting a long time, the Flatheads had gone home empty-handed, and only when the northwestern wilderness had covered their tracks did American Christendom cry shame upon itself. The first to respond were the Methodists, who sent their own mission around the Horn to settle in the virgin paradise of the Willamette Valley. The pique of this must have been in the mind of the Congregational Doctor Greene and the Board as they pondered Whitman's application. More, the American public was crying that something must be done about the flat heads of the Flatheads — in spite of the fact that this tribe, which calls itself the Salish, do not flatten their heads and are misnamed by their white brothers. Perhaps that is why Marcus Whitman, M.D., was at last permitted to go to the assistance of these stultified people, with the blessing of the Board and a sum of money which strained its funds to the limit.

But he did not go alone. The Reverend Henry H. Spalding and his wife Eliza volunteered for this perilous labor of grace. And the young doctor had found, on his return from Wyoming, a sweetheart already determined on a missionary's career. She was Miss Narcissa Prentiss of Amity, New York, daughter of a judge and sister, by temperament, to suffering mankind. She had some time ago rejected the suit of the Reverend Henry Spalding, whom Eliza consoled, and it is likely that, with her wealth of fair hair, her sweet blue eyes, her prime young figure and lilting voice, she had had many opportunities to embrace a tranquil and happy fate. Instead she chose a path which no white woman had ever gone before — the Oregon Trail, on the trip that first broke it.

There was still the late spring snow of 1836 upon the gentle hills of central York state when 'Husband,' as she called him, tucked his bride of the flowerlike name into the sleigh and drove her away from the home that she would never see again. Behind them, inured to any weather, speaking only with their big black eyes or in crowlike syllables, rode the two Nez Percé Indian boys, Ais and Tackitooitis.

Western travel, Narcissa discovered, is divided and classified by what you have to eat. The first stage is the one supplied by the stores you can carry with you; the next is the buffalo zone, with the smell of new kill roasting; the third and worst is the jerk-meat period, when you try to swallow dirty salted leather and praise God for it — God and a husband who had learned to cook it, who could find fuel where there was no fuel, and fresh water where others, even the Indian boys, knew only foul.

It was in this stage of their westward progress that the young people, all but Whitman tenderfeet, crossed the Continental Divide through the South Pass — both brides pregnant and Mrs. Spalding vomiting and fainting — and came down on the lush grass of the old Green River rendezvous. All knelt down; one man held the Bible, another the American flag, and, in their own words, they took possession of this wilderness as the home of future American mothers and the church of a merciful Jesus.

Under the great empty dome that roofs Wyoming, shots rang out. There was a wild yelling such as Indians make; balls whistled over the heads of the travelers, and in an instant the missionaries were surrounded by a crazy crew of white men brown as savages and twice as frenzied. They rode around, Narcissa wrote back to her gentle mother and sisters, like mad men; they seized the hands of the two wives and pumped them to breaking. Some of these grizzled Mountain Men wept, for they had not seen a white woman since they crossed the Mississippi five, ten, or twenty years before. The first white women ever to come over the Rockies! That word flew from mouth to mouth; the news was ridden off in every direction, and every hour more men born of women came galloping up, to catch off their hats and fill their eyes. The Flatheads and the Nez Percés, the Shoshones and Bannocks, looked on with obsidian eyes which no one thought to try to read. But the squaws took charge of Mrs. Spalding; they knew all about her trouble and they fed her certain roots they dug, and fresh trout instead of jerky. And from then on, both wives were strong again.

Then the wagons once more rolled forward, crushing the sage that never before had bent to a wheel. Beyond this there were mountains like walls and canyons like cracks in the floor of hell; beyond this no axle would ever creak, declared Bridger and Fitzpatrick and Donald McKay, the Whitmans' guide. But the young doctor struck the air with the bullhide whip, and the oxen strained forward over the rocks. If he had to take his wagons apart, Whitman swore, and carry the wheels on his shoulders, he would still get through to set those wheels to rolling down the Pacific slope. The white man's wheel, the white man's woman, the white man's God, he would take them to Oregon, and set them there in honor.

The wheel could not speak, and the God did not need to, but Narcissa wrote what it was like to go west with Marcus Whitman:

> I have such a good place to shelter — under my husband's wings. He is so excellent. I love to confide in his judgment and act under him. He is just like mother in telling me of my failings. He does it in such a way that I like to have him, for it gives me a chance to improve.

She was a bride, you may say, in the first blinding transports of wedded love, but everything we hear about Whitman tells us how big a man he was. He had a crackling hearthfire of a heart; there seemed to be nothing for which he was not strong enough; there was no number of things, you'd say, he could not do at once. He perfectly fulfilled the old phrase about being all things to all men. He was a man among the cultivated, a gentleman even with savages, an adored father to all children, and in Narcissa's arms he was 'Husband.' He could mend, with strips of oxhide from the beasts that died on the way, the shrunken rims of the wagon wheels. When the axles smoked with strain, he would scrape pitch from the pines to grease them; he healed with tar the bleeding feet of the beasts; he knew, Narcissa wrote, a different way of cooking every kind of meat. He could get frightened animals to swim, and weary women to laughing.

The hardest part of the trip was the last, through the wildest wilderness of Idaho and eastern Oregon. It was better, though, as far as food went; the Indian boys caught salmon in the streams and dug sweet camas roots from the boggy meadows where the deer fled them. There was deer meat and elk meat, and Narcissa dined on mutton from the Rocky Mountain sheep. In many ways it was easier or at least much pleasanter to be the first white woman in the West than the ten thousandth, for in those days sixty thousand immigrants had not passed ahead of you, killing off the game in every direction, their cattle cutting the range grasses to the root, polluting the streams, clouding with dust the bright western horizon. Nor had the reasonable fears and resentments of the Indians been roused as yet. These first-comers could actually count upon Indian aid. They voyaged, God-fearing, through an Eden of elk and moose, muskrat, mink, and beaver, of twinkling aspens and hushing fir and spruce; under the August sun the earth rendered up its breath of rosin and bracken, lichen and warm, dry needles — pure and living as a deer's.

Then on a day, after a toilsome ascent of the Blue Mountains, they looked down upon the vast valley of the Columbia. A hundred miles away to the west rose the Cascade Range, topped by its extinct volcanoes. These are our seven Fujiyamas, truncated cones capped with the snows that are brought them by the damp Pacific winds. The sunset light was in the travelers' eyes as they rode out upon the valley slopes; it burnished the wild rye grass. The Indians called this *waiilatpu* 'place of rye grass.' Where rye grass will grow, Whitman reasoned, wheat will grow; the seed grain in the little sack he had brought was the white man's bread coming with the white man's God.

So it was there that the Whitmans founded their mission, calling it Waiilatpu. The Spaldings went a hundred and twenty miles northeastward, among the Nez Percés, to found Lapwai on the Clearwater. The Nez Percés urged Whitman, too, to come amongst them. Those Cayuse around you, they said, are bad Indians; they are ungrateful and treacherous. Some day you will see.

The farther off they are from God, Whitman answered, the more they need us. And he planted his apple trees, he plowed his ground and sowed his wheat, and the Lord blessed his cattle and his flocks so that they multiplied and grew fat. And when he had raised his house, Narcissa's time was come upon her. This had long been a matter of speculation among the Indians, and they seemed to know better than she the appointed day. So that a multitude was gathered at the mission, all wishing to be present at the miraculous event. When the child was born, her mother named her Alice Clarissa, but the Indians called her 'Cayuse Girl.' And grim chiefs picked up her hand, frail as a windflower, in dark, curious fingers.

'I fear I love her too well,' Narcissa wrote home. Even the Cayuse were proud of her, this first-born Oregonian. But there was a dark current that ran through Waiilatpu. Whitman had built upon the banks of the Walla Walla; children cannot leave water alone, and they do not understand its depth. The curly-haired two-year-old wanted only enough of the river to fill her two small cups. Instead, the river took her. It was an old Indian who dived many times to recover her body, and he laid it at last with a genuine and profound sorrow upon the bank.

With the child's death ended the morning of Narcissa's adventure; and perhaps something was never quite the same again between the Indians and the Whitmans after Cayuse Girl died. The red men had considered her part of their tribe and, as Narcissa never had another child, the Whitmans again became foreigners.

The ideal of the Protestant missionary is to set an example of the white man's way of life, to teach it and spread it. That nothing is harder to do well, thousands of miles from the white man's culture and among a people in the New Stone Age, must not deter the missionary from devotion to his task. But when Whitman plowed the earth, which is the red man's mother, it seemed to the Cayuse that he was desecrating divine flesh. For these were not a planting people, but fish-eating Indians. They said that damp vapors came out of the plowed ground, and gave them inflammation of the lungs, as punishment for this white man's temerity. They did not like the example of Christian family life. During Narcissa's pregnancy Marcus cooked and swept and did the washing, like a good American husband in a domestic pinch. A fine fix the Cayuse would have been in, if they had become the slaves of their squaws like that! It was obvious to them that if only Narcissa had done the plowing and developed the habit of carrying a full water jug on her head as she walked, she would have had the baby easily, and many others.

The democracy of Christianity was repugnant to the chiefs; if there were any benefits to be had from this new medicine called the Word of God, it should have been revealed secretly, they felt, to themselves as élite. When Narcissa adopted an orphan Cayuse boy, a hideous old squaw, with no one to look out for her, presented herself and her fleas for adoption as well. The word 'adoption' means two different things to these two races of Americans, and the squaw went away embittered by Christian hypocrisy. But it does not take an Indian long to discover charity where charity is; the vegetables and milk, the butter and apples of Waiilatpu, its mutton and hams, its eggs and pullets, were assumed to be the fruits of conversion. However much you gave the converts, they came back for more.

As for Christian ceremony, the Cayuse could never get enough of that, either. They sang hymns gladly, both at the mission and among themselves; they loved to hear Bible stories — the serpent and the first squaw, the old chief that took the animals into his big canoe, the girl that cut off the warrior's hair so that his enemies slew him. Word of these stories passed through the forests, and savages came and sat rows deep to hear this entertainment.

But when Whitman upbraided them for their sloth and gluttony, when he called them dirty, thieving, lying — which they so abundantly were — when he hurled the terrible Commandments at their heads, when he cut through their genial mysticism with the ice and fire of Christ's own words, their feelings at first were merely injured. 'Do not tell us we are not good Christians,' they begged him, disgruntled. 'Do not ask us to do these hard things which no one does. Do not use such bad language to us.' They were being most forbearing with him — for Cayuse — since to upbraid an Indian is the same as to strike him. With time their forbearance ebbed, and deep resentment flooded to take its place. Whitman fed them when they were hungry and clothed them when they were naked and healed them when they were sick. And something troubled them like a light that they could not endure with their eyes, so that they crawled away into the dark places that had so long been familiar to them.

Beside the zeal of a man of God, Whitman had the physician's professional code, nor did he deviate from it. He answered every call, and though he had just come in from a distant journey, he would, if summoned, lift his weary body onto a fresh mount and ride off in another direction, to set a bone or treat a desperate case of scarlet fever, trepan a skull, or ease the dying. There were the Methodists, more than a hundred miles away in the Willamette Valley; they sent for him so often and he came so many times that he began to build a road between their station and his! There were the Hudson's Bay men and their *voyageurs*, French Canadians and halfbreeds — they had their share of ailments. There were the missions to the east and north, and the immigrant trains that had now begun to come.

And always there were the Indians. They called their own doctors *te-wats*, medicine men; to them Whitman was just another *te-wat* subject to the same ethical code, namely, death at the hands of the outraged relatives if a patient died in his care. Over and over he was threatened with this vengeance. He had to forbid Narcissa to administer even tincture of arnica to little bruises. For himself, he never flinched. He took all risks.

The Indians were not Whitman's only troubles. One of a missionary's crosses is other missionaries, and other sects, and the good people at home who do not know what he's up against. The correspondence of Marcus Whitman and the Reverend Doctor David Greene fills a fat published volume; we should look with some pity on the efforts of the Secretary of the Board to see as far as from Cornhill to Walla Walla. Books on secular subjects, anvils, flower seeds, improved plows, drugs — these requisitions on the slender funds of the Board it could not understand, back in Boston. Greene seems trying hard to back Brother Whitman in his novel endeavors, but the effort is too much for him, and he usually closes his letters by raising his eyes and hands to heaven.

For out in Oregon the mission had almost lost sight of its original purpose — the making of good Protestants out of bad Cayuse. The Board had never visualized Waiilatpu as a restaurant, wrote the unhappy Secretary. It was more; it had developed into a hotel at which several hundred immigrants a year arrived weary and famished and were allowed to stay as long as they found necessary. It had become a public school, with between fifty and eighty children boarded and taught here; Mountain Men like Joe Meek and Jim Bridger sent their daughters to it with a sigh of relief at getting them in Narcissa Whitman's hands. Waiilatpu was an orphanage too; what was Narcissa to do when the Sager boy of seventeen, his parents having died on the Oregon Trail, drove a wagon to the door bringing six other little Sagers, the baby with a broken leg? The place was a hospital, of course, and a maternity home; on occasion it was an asylum for the mentally ill — at least one of the missionaries went quite insane and, there being no way to send him home, he was tended for a year in this crowded house of good will. Naturally, Waiilatpu was also a fort, though it was hard for the Board to see why Whitman wanted firearms and ammunition when he had gone out to save souls. Also, it was a vast cooperative farm and self-supporting plantation. And, with her husband, Narcissa held the reins of the whole enterprise.

In the midst of their labors, there arrived at Waiilatpu a letter from the Board coolly closing this mission to the unpromising Cayuse. It was more important — so it appeared on Cornhill — to further the blessed work among the Sandwich Islanders. As for the American immigrants whose feet Whitman was binding up, Doctor Greene opined that such men as would leave the intellectual refinements of the East for western barbarity would be of 'very little good to Oregon.' And closing his letter of command to Marcus Whitman, he signed himself, 'Very truly your servant in Christ.'

But Whitman had long since ceased to be primarily a sectarian missionary, nor was he merely a doctor now. He had become a prophet of the opening West, and Narcissa saw his true prevision with him. All the other Americans who came out when he first came considered themselves sojourners; Marcus Whitman was the first Oregonian. In God's name he and his wife had knelt to claim this land for our flag and our way, and here they had borne and buried their seed.

Not yet had Horace Greeley exclaimed, 'Go West, young man!' In fact, he was — for party purposes — opposing western migration. He would have been flabbergasted if he could have heard that inside of seventeen years the Governor of Oregon would be a candidate for Vice-President of the United States. But this would have astonished Whitman not at all, I think. Six years of riding Oregon convinced him that America had, in the Northwest, a sparkling empire for the conquering.

Yet her light grasp upon it was slipping. The rival claims of Canada to the territory had been admitted when the United States signed an agreement with Great Britain for joint occupancy of the country. Under these terms both peoples might settle there, neither with jurisdiction over the other. This seems square enough, if perilous with seeds of controversy, but the British settlers had a great advantage in the Hudson's Bay Company's system of fortified trading posts. The Company represented a powerful network of unified interest; it was in a position, as the British immigrant's banker, grocer, and buyer, to pass him along from post to post, and to safeguard him wherever he went; Company rules and discipline were a sort of law out in a lawless land. The American, on the other hand, could appeal to no sort of authority. The writ of the United States did not run this far; in Oregon a settler could not bequeath or inherit, he could not sue, or appeal for protection to any court. He had no friends but the missionaries. And now if Waiilatpu, at the very gate of Oregon, was to be closed out, then the overland door would be shut to the searching current of American growth. In this way Oregon inevitably would become British — unless that door to it were swept open and kept open.

All this Marcus Whitman laid before his fellow workers, and proposed to ride East to waken the country. The brethren shook doubtful heads. Let him stick to preaching the Word of God, and leave politics alone! Whitman got to his feet, his hands making passionate fists before him, and told them all: 'I was a man before I became a missionary, and when I became a missionary I did not expatriate myself. I shall go to the States if I have to sever my connection with the mission.' So that's how he kissed Narcissa good-bye, that autumn of 1842, mounted his horse, and rode toward the ranges, toward winter's gales and snows, and the cold of Eastern lethargy.

He broke new paths through the mountains, and in places even his guides turned back. Supporting himself alone in the ice-locked wilderness, Marcus Whitman rode on, steadily, wearily, pushing his horse as hard as he dared and himself harder. In funds he was very low; his old fur cap was worn to the skin and his buffalo coat whipped raggedly in the wind; the heavy beard was graying now; the big hands, that had slapped the breath into babies and baptized savage heads and felled timbers and planted trees, shook the bridle for more haste.

Men in the farthest outposts saw unbelieving this snow-covered wraith appear out of the West. Old Mountain Men turned and stared at his shouted greeting. Not since the return of Lewis and Clark over thirty years ago had St. Louis beheld so seasoned a returned traveler. He made all speed across the slush and ice of March in the eastern states, going straight to the Secretary of War in Washington, to lay before him the Oregon situation. Then to Greeley in New York to make clear to the publicist his vision of the West. And at last he came striding into the meeting room of the shocked Board of Missions on Cornhill in Boston.

When he entered that room, he had every circumstance and every member against him. When he left it, he had converted even these pious men to saving the Oregon missions.

So he turned back west, for the tide of settlers he had prophesied was already rising, promising to flood the British claims out of the Oregon country — if they could get through to it. They *must* get through, and Whitman undertook to pilot them in person. It was he who knew the water holes and the grass and the passes, he who could support the weary and mend the broken. Some he buried, many he delivered, more he saved; now, as always, whenever Doctor Whitman appeared, the way eased and the heart lifted. His early dream of rolling a wagon wheel up and over the Rockies came true now in giant proportion. And that this phantom wheel bearing a thousand pioneering Americans ever achieved the Continental Divide and passed it, was in great measure because one man put so stout a shoulder to it.

The emigrants settled like locusts upon Waiilatpu; in a few days they had cleaned it of the stores of years, in their desperate need, till there was nothing left to eat but some immature potatoes under ground. Waiilatpu, and its master and mistress, undoubtedly saved the first and most crucial wave to come over the Oregon Trail. And it was the presence of this American advance which, soon after, was to cause Britain to give up as hopeless its claims to our Northwest.

But the Cayuse correctly read their doom in this irresistible invasion. Faster ran the dark current through Waiilatpu. One man they blamed, with a justice of their own. And, as just as they, Whitman himself admitted that the cause of his red children was lost; they would not be saved, and he could not save them.

When a brave woman is frightened, she is more defiantly brave than ever. To read Narcissa's letters home is to hear always the undercurrent of that dark river running through her home, rising a little more each night, bearing down from wilder places the sound that every Westerner feared, of ruthless waters caught between unyielding walls.

Yet by day the Walla Walla sparkled placidly; the Cayuse came and went; they still sang hymns, they still gulped obediently the medicine poured them. And there was much of this, because measles had come west with the pale-faces, and this disease, new to the Cayuse, struck old and young alike in a form as deadly as smallpox. To an Indian every disease is caused by the malevolence of something or somebody. It was a logical deduction for the Cayuse to assume that the sickness which appeared with Whitman's reappearance was not cured by him because he had resolved upon the destruction of the tribe.

So they said that he was poisoning them, and to ignorant people the whisper of poison acts like the cry of fire among crowded people. When now their oldest friends among the Cayuse became disaffected, the Whitmans felt the ground going out from under their feet. Now their converts neither came to the mission nor yet left its neighborhood, but stood about at a little distance and watched the mission people bring out their dead and bury them. And Marcus and Narcissa looked at each other and then looked quickly away again, lest the eyes of the children should intercept their glance.

The enemies of a physician know that his weak point is that he can refuse no calls. When a Cayuse named Young Chief came on Saturday afternoon, November 27, 1847, asking the doctor to come to his village, Whitman had no choice but to go. Above all he must show no sign of fear, lest he have up the whole wolf pack. Through the rain and fog he rode away, and at Young Chief's village he found two newly come Jesuit fathers, baptizing the babies and burying the dying. Since the priests never attempted much medical healing, they were not in conflict with the *te-wats*, not resented by the Cayuse, and all unconscious of the rising hatred of these Indians for Whitman. So they were astonished to find the doctor agitated, and surprised at the warmth with which he urged them to come to visit at Waiilatpu, without fail, tomorrow if possible. They did not hear that this big, strong, brave man was begging them for whatever influence to peace they might bring upon the savages ringing his station.

Through the darkness and the blowing mists the doctor rode back, and no one will ever know what dread was in his heart. But when he reached 'the place of rye grass,' the dawn light showed him the schoolhouse, the mansion house, the dormitories, the mill, the blacksmith shop, all standing tranquilly in the soft cold air. That last Sunday at Waiilatpu began quietly, wearily, for there were many sick in the house. But Narcissa did not touch her breakfast, and they found her weeping.

Yet, come terror or tragedy, meals must be cooked and babies washed and all the other small domestic rites performed as long as possible. In such domestic business the afternoon opened. Then there was a knock on the door. Narcissa, coming out of the pantry with milk for the children, saw two blanketed figures at the kitchen door; the doctor admitted them into the house. A gunshot rang out, and a moment later Jim Bridger's little girl rushed screaming in to Narcissa. She had seen the doctor tomahawked from behind, and the Sager boy shot.

The shot was a prearranged signal; all over the ranch little knots of infiltrating Indians had stationed themselves strategically. At the blacksmith shop they cut down some of the whites; in the open spaces between buildings they concentrated their fire on any who attempted to gain shelter. They smashed in the doors, and they hunted in every corner to track down all the men. There was then no one left for them to fear but Mrs. Whitman, the woman who had the evil white *te-wat's* medicine in her. And they shot at her through a window, wounding her, but still she kept her feet, kept her control of the terrified children, whom she hastened away upstairs under lock and key.

But the Indians threatened the house with fire; they warned her to come out, and offered a parley. There was nothing to do but accept their proposal; descending, Narcissa came, at the foot of the stairs, upon her husband's mutilated body, and fainted away. So she was carried out into the open, and there, in easy range of a waiting Cayuse squad, under the Oregon sky, she took a short leaden death to her breast.

Those who were killed, the priests came to bury. Those who were captured were ransomed after a month of slavery. The Cayuse were driven from their lands, and the ringleaders of the massacre delivered up to justice and dispatched out of this world. Now the Oregon Trail rang to the tread of United States troops marching to establish law and order on the land that the Whitmans had consecrated with their blood. Now there could be no question that this land was and must remain wholly American. The Whitmans' was not only a religious martyrdom, and death in the great name of medical healing; they died for their country too. However dreadful the short passage by which they left this world, theirs was the glory of giving their lives for all they held most dear.

16

Mr. Carson and the Indians

THERE IS ALWAYS GOLD in the West; in every sunset the simplest child can see it. The early Spanish explorers of our Southwest marched and countermarched in quest of it. They came to the shores where the sun goes down, and still they had not found it. We'd have to say that they weren't very good prospectors; they wanted to rely on Indians who might be possessed of gold; their plan was to find whoever had it and take it away from them. The more civilized Indians of Mexico and Peru had the ductile metal and knew how to work it; so they became the Spaniards' first victims. But the Indians of North America, of the Far West, were spirits free of the idolatry of gold. They saw pure lumps of the stuff gleaming in the river sands, and it did not bewitch them. You see, they were too stupid to wash the mountains open to get more of this yellow dust, and they were too brute ignorant to kill each other for a claim upon it. What they gladly killed for was a claim that ran deeper than any vein.

And now, in the miraculous year of Forty-Nine, the white men were coming to dispute that claim. Along the Santa Fé Trail the Apaches were waiting for them. Their first victims were the party of a wealthy merchant, going west to trade in the little Spanish capital. One boy alone escaped, and what he told in Taos sent Major Grier off at a gallop with his dragoons. For the Apaches had carried off the merchant's wife alive.

Official guide of the rescue expedition was one Leroux, cocksure he knew all Injun ways, green-jealous of a soft-mannered man who had ridden over to help, from his ranch near Wagon Mound. This fellow was undersized, which made him appear ineffective. His eyes looked mild as a kitten's. Speaking seldom, swearing less, he never raised his voice. Men who did not live long enough to acknowledge their mistake had sometimes taken this for effeminacy.

Unlike Leroux, he didn't boast. Following Apache, he warned, was like hunting quail; they scatter, leaving you fifty tracks to choose from. All looked alike to the worried Major. But the wiry little man unraveled the trail of the Apaches as a hound goes after a fox upwind. He was quick but wary, so cautious that he showed the Major the whole Indian camp before its sharpest sentinel spied them. Now was the moment to attack! But Leroux overrode him; the Major delayed an hour, and the dragoons were discovered. So quickly and secretly did the redskins break camp that the soldiers never got a shot. All that was left them was the murdered body of the merchant's wife.

In her pathetic baggage the remorseful Major found a book, a dime thriller about a fellow named Kit Carson. They handed the mild little man his biography, but Mr. Carson shook his head. 'They laid it on a leetle thick,' said he.

For even while he lived, Kit was a legend. Yet many of the most fabulous of his escapes were true; an Apache bullet *did* pass through his hair; a badman's rifle *was* fired so close the powder burned Kit's cheek. Ambushed by fifty Comanches, he dashed through a hail of missiles unscathed. Winged by Blackfeet, unable then to shoot, he had to dodge from tree to tree, and that night sleep without fire in the snow — which probably stopped the bleeding and so saved his life. Attacked once by a huge bear, he was busy with old Bruin when Mrs. Grizzly came roaring up behind him; Kit came home with both skins. Commissioned to ride a message for help through hostile Ute country, he took a pal, Sol Silver, with him. When the Utes tracked them, Sol told Kit to go ahead with the letter and the faster horse. Kit started, but when he saw the Utes coming for old Sol he rode back. 'We'll get rubbed out together,' Sol reports him as saying. But the savages, recognizing what man they had to deal with, decided that fifty to two were odds too unfavorable.

Men said he led a charmed life, but Kit's magic was simply an accurate knowledge of Indian ways. As a guide on a pursuit of murderous Jicarillas, he told his commanding officer he calculated from sign they'd come up with the foe at two that afternoon. Major Carleton admired Mr. Carson, but doubted so bold a prediction; he bet a hat his guide was wrong. Yet when scouts signaled 'enemy in sight' the Major consulted his timepiece. Two, to the tick! That's how a *genuwine* beaver hat came all the way from the States, inscribed, 'At Two O'Clock. Kit Carson, from Major Carleton.'

These are not legends but facts acknowledged even by Kit's enemies, or extracted from sober army reports. William Tecumseh Sherman recorded: 'They seem to think out here that Carson's a bigger man than I am, and they seem to be right. His integrity is simply perfect.' Frémont wrote, 'With me Carson and Truth are one.' So the truth becomes greater than the legend. Kit Carson was no mere Indian fighter; he was a natural gentleman, a fine diplomat, and the greatest of all American guides, who held open for the first wagon trains the door to California.

Christopher Carson came of simple stock, the same sort that produced Boone and Lincoln. His father, from the redhill country of North Carolina, married Rebecca Robinson and by her had ten children — Kit the fifth of them. When one year old, he was taken to Missouri. Not far away from the sandy-haired baby, Dan Boone was eating out his heart because he was too old to explore the Rockies, and morosely building himself a coffin. Boone it was who had led white settlement to the Mississippi; where he left off, Carson took up. No one man in history had more to do with adding to our country that vast area, larger than the rebellious Confederacy which Lincoln brought back to the Union — the old Southwest. Those words ring with the excitement of stagecoaches and army posts, gold rushes and Conestogas, the golden spike and the trampling herds. But these came after Kit; he made these possible. Pre-railroad, pre-stagecoach, pre-cowboy, Kit went ahead and found a way, through hunger, thirst, and tribes of blood-lusty Indians.

When Kit was fifteen, a falling tree killed Pappy Carson; unwillingly the boy took his seat at an apprentice saddle-maker's bench, in the raw town of Franklin, Missouri. That was a great outfitting post for the western caravans. And here a company of fur-trappers came, to get their gear all ship-shape; it was none less than old Bent himself, of Bent, St. Vrain and Company, who gave Kit a knee up. For the lad slipped away from his saddler's bench, and the hard-bitten Mountain Men, trekking west again, grinned down at the sawed off, skinny youngster, all freckles and sandy mop, toting Pappy's rusty flintlock longer than himself. Back in Franklin, the master saddler advertised sardonically for his runaway apprentice — reward one cent.

But Kit was off for the West he had dreamed of; he was 'cavvy,' the wrangler who has the mean job of rounding up the lazy or foal-heavy stragglers at the rear. In 'Santy Fee' and Taos, Kit learned cooking, teamstering, gun-mending, bullet-running, and, from the señoritas, Spanish. He rode the Santa Fé Trail a year and more, hating the eastward trip, loving the westbound. Then he tried the California haul, and killed his first redskin, with a bull's-eye to the heart. That was when he drove his first brass tack in his gunstock. For each man killed in a face-to-face fight, he drove another tack. After eighteen of them he gave up count.

When young Kit blew into Taos again, he was mounted and rich, a full-fledged Mountain Man, with fur collar, brass buttons, velvet insertions, and locks of the girls of Los Angeles pueblo tied to the fringes of his leggings. His wealth lasted a week. When mule and silver-mounted saddle and spurs were gone, he joined the Rocky Mountain trappers.

For those were the glory days of the fur trade, when the dictates of male fashion decreed that every Eastern gentleman must wear a beaver hat. So for the hide of the little flat-tailed wilderness engineer, men of the stamp of Jim and Gabe Bridger, Charles and William Bent, Sublette, St. Vrain, Colter, and Gaunt worked country a thousand miles from any army post, daring Montana Blackfeet, Utah Apaches, all the fiercest tribes of the West.

After ten years of this, Carson knew every inch of the Rockies from Montana to New Mexico. As plains and desert had made of him an expert horseman, teamster, saddler, gun-mender, bullet-runner, and buffalo hunter, so the mountains and forests taught him to make snowshoes, build canoes and bullboats. He learned French as Canadian halfbreeds speak it, Mexican Spanish, Arapaho, Comanche, Cheyenne, Ute, and the universal sign language. He could identify hoofmarks not only of his own horses but those of many another well-known Westerner, of red men, badmen, Mountain Men. From a moccasin print he could tell of what tribe was the Indian who passed. He could judge the sex, age, height or weight, and usually the state of mind of the maker of any footstep.

Where even old Gaunt could find no beaver, Kit trapped behind him and got a fortune in pelts. He was saving money now, organizing his own fur business. He had his pick of the best trappers of his time and he chose an outfit that became known as 'The Carson Men.' They formed a nucleus of rough and ready law in a disorganized society, and were noted for their honesty and courage. As a fighting unit far ahead of the army, they were formidable. Two hundred Blackfeet backed down when Kit entrenched his men before them. That was when the Indians began to call him 'Little Chief.'

Spring was on the sage of the Green River country when Little Chief rode down out of the Wyoming mountains and saw Waa-nibe, Singing Grass, dancing the spoon dance among the Mountain Men. She was fresh in her teens, in only her bright skirt; there were modesty and goodness in her dark Arapaho eyes. But one of the men, who had no respect for the ritual of the dance, and less for any squaw, tried to force her. Kit shot him down in front of the whole camp. That night Kit walked into Waa-nibe's tepee and sat beside her. She was peeling with her teeth the willow rods to weave a bridal bed. And her father rose and laid his blanket ceremonially over the shoulders of his daughter and Little Chief.

Kit called her Alice, and no squaw had ever been treated like that before. She was loaded with presents, taken everywhere Kit went, mounted on a fine horse, presently with her papoose on her back. Kit named their child Adaline, the sweet. In 1839 Kit came back from a great buffalo hunt and found Singing Grass dying. Medicine men were beating the drum, trying by its rhythm to slow her rising pulse, but the drums of her heart flew faster and faster; she died in Kit's arms. He saw her marriage bed burned, and her dresses; her brother shot her dog and horse to accompany her on her lonely way. Amid the din of ceremonial Indian mourning, Little Chief, terror of the Sioux and Apache, bowed his head.

But Waa-nibe, Alice Singing Grass, in her short life accomplished much. From her in great part Carson learned to understand the red brother, and to respect him. 'A brave man,' he would say of some savage who had defied him, 'but he barred the wrong passage.' Carson came to comprehend what was honor to an Indian; he could read the stone face. He made of friendlier tribes his allies, used them as scouts and hunters; to catch a Comanche he learned to set a Jicarilla. His wife taught him pity for the fate of these wilderness princes who defended their lands against the inevitable march of white civilization.

With courage to match his sympathy, Kit Carson yet never

provoked an Indian attack, never fired on squaws or let the
Carson Men do so. But when the redskins raided the whites,
he knew how to punish them. If it came to a fight he was
both intrepid and careful. Even when defeated he could be
victorious. In the Texas Panhandle, at the battle of Adobe
Walls, with four hundred men he was surrounded by five thousand Plains Indians; his situation for a while was much like
Custer's on the banks of the Little Bighorn. But unlike that
West Point tactician, Carson did not divide his forces and
fatally attack an enemy of unknown strength. When the
Indians fired the grass Carson backfired it, and cut his way out
of an overwhelming encirclement; he did what all commanders find hardest, in retreat kept his force intact and unhurried, reversing his supply trains without confusion.

'The prettiest fight I ever saw,' Kit used to call a hot brush
with the Indians. But he loved the ways of peace too. In old
Taos with its clashing bells and smell of pinyon smoke, its patio
gardens and secretive Spanish houses, and its motley crowd of
Indians, Spaniards, traders, trappers, and adventurers of all
colors, Kit was always happiest, and Taos formed the setting
of his last and greatest romance. The lady, Señorita Maria
Josefa Jaramillo, is said to have had a 'haughty, heartbreaking
beauty.' She was fifteen when they married, and Christopher
was thirty-four. She was sheltered and high-born; he was
weathered by exposure to life. But she knew a man when she
met one. Never haughty with Kit, this heartbreaker took care
of that tough and tender thing, the heart of Christopher Carson.

Before his marriage, he took Adaline to the nuns in Missouri. On the way back he met a dashing lieutenant, one
John Charles Frémont, then the newest of tenderfeet, who was
starting out to explore the passes of the Rockies for his government. Carson he hired as guide, and there sprang up a
friendship that never died. Poles apart, these two complemented each other perfectly. Frémont was highly cultivated,
dashing, reckless, ambitious, subtle in the politics of army and

Washington intrigue, and Kit admired every inch of him. Frémont returned the admiration; his reports of Kit made Carson famous in the East, from farm to city street. But Carson carried Frémont to fame, too, by showing him the way through the Rockies; Frémont's report on the passes made the Mormon trek possible, and opened the Overland Trail for the Forty-Niners' covered wagons.

Kit guided Frémont on his first three and greatest expeditions, over thousands of unmapped miles, from water hole to water hole, through the stratagems of Indian fighting and the tricks of Spanish diplomacy, and led Frémont's guns to Sutter's Fort before ever General Kearney, officially appointed to take California, had left Texas.

Kit galloped east with news of the victory for the White House. But in New Mexico he met Kearney, poking along with his infantry. The General took the letters and gave them to another messenger to deliver, commandeering Carson to guide him. Nearing San Diego, Kearney ordered an advance right into a Mexican trap, was beaten, surrounded, and cut off from water. Messenger after messenger was sent by the beleaguered general for help from the American garrison at San Diego. Not one got through. Then Kit offered to go.

All night, down with the rattlesnakes and cactus, he crawled on his belly through the Mexican lines. When he stood up at dawn he found that his shoes, tied to his back, had been wrenched off in the brush. He walked barefoot daylong over the cruelest of deserts, crept all night again through another enemy ring, until he heard the challenge of the Yankee sentries. This time Kit was allowed the honor due him, of carrying the news to Washington. There President Polk handed him a commission in the army. But Kearney's jealous intrigues caused Congress to refuse to confirm it. For his two years' service with Frémont, Kit Carson was not allowed a cent of pay.

Back in Taos, Kit was ready to settle down. In six years he had had only sixteen months with his young wife. And he had plans and visions. The old fur trade was going; silk hats had sprung the beaver traps. Moreover, the buffalo were vanishing, and the days of easy meat. So Carson went into ranching, and became one of the earliest cowboys in the West. Settlers were pouring in now, and he bred horses and raised mules for them. Decades before the herders came, Kit saw the value in mutton and wool, and drove sixty-five hundred head of sheep from New Mexico through a country infested with coyotes and Indians to San Francisco, where he made a fine profit on them. The old Indian fighter was showing the way to Western prosperity through the industries of peace. And a wise government now made him Indian agent at Taos.

Christopher Carson was the greatest Indian diplomatist in history. By his understanding of the red men he saved more lives and won more square miles than by all his fifty pitched battles with them. Unable himself to read or write, he knew better than to make a paper treaty with a savage who would sign his mark to anything and change his mind next day, with no sense of lost honor. The Indian had his own code, and Kit comprehended it. Called on to guide a military company to overtake and punish the Jicarillas, he found that the soldiers had captured a friendly Ute, taken his gun away from him and tied him up. In the night the Ute escaped. When Kit heard of it, he saw what that would mean — a Ute-Jicarilla axis to face. He took the dangerous gun and rode hard for Taos, where he sent out messages to the Ute chiefs to come and see him, and at his mere request they rode in, a hundred and two hundred miles. After he had feasted them and given them presents, he returned the gun. The soldiers have made a mistake, he said, and Uncle Sam apologizes.

For, his life long, Kit never cheated a savage. He was disgusted with the way white traders got Indians drunk and then robbed them. As Indian agent, he did much to undo the effects produced by other whites when they robbed, kicked, flogged, and insulted Indians, shot them on sight, seduced their girls, and stole their lands. The red men came to call him 'Father Kit.'

Aged early by hardship, saddened by the death of Josefa in childbirth, he found himself in failing health. Yet, sick and suffering, he stood by his Indian charges and went all the way to Washington with a delegation of Ute chiefs who wished to appeal to the President. At Fort Lyon, on the return, a doctor was called in. He shook his head; Mr. Carson might live some time — on a diet of milksop.

Kit gave him a look, from those mild blue eyes. Then he called in his servant from the kitchen. 'Cook me some fust-rate doin's,' he said. 'Buffalo steak, strong coffee, and a pipe of tobacco is what I need to fix me.'

Inevitably, hemorrhage followed this Mountain Man's meal. 'I'm gone!' Kit exulted. 'Doctor, *compadre*, *adios!*'

They buried General Christopher Carson in the bleak Plains cemetery of old Fort Lyon, with full military honors. Spring hadn't really got to Colorado by May 23 of 1868; at least, there weren't enough flowers to lay on his grave, so the women of the army post gave the paper posies out of their hats. Later his remains were carried to Taos, and laid there beside his beloved Josefa, in holy ground. But Kit had blessed with new security more ground than any churchyard could hold — eight hundred thousand square miles of it, where the American wind goes whispering about him, through the pinyon and the mesquite.

All Americans know Kit Carson stories, the way they know Boone and Bridger stories. The explorer and scout, the Indian fighter and the first man to do this or that, is the favorite hero of a people who have always been proud to get there ahead of the rest. With us, the scout is more beloved than the purely military hero; you praise a man heartily when you dub him 'a good scout.' That means he'll stand by you if you're in trouble and, if it comes to that, he'll get rubbed out along of you, before he'll leave you. It means he sees his way ahead, and will lead those who depend on him. It means he'll fight it out only if that's what it has come to, and fight clean. And for American boys like mine there is no pledge more binding than 'Scout's honor.'

Most of our early scouts were Indian-fighters, I've said, but their most typical traits and much of their resourcefulness were copied from the Indians. 'Go,' says an old Apache chief today, to the young men drafted off the reservation to fight in North Africa and the East Indies, 'go and conduct yourselves like brave scouts.' For to be a brave scout and a good one occupies the same place of honor among red Americans as among the white; nor did they learn that from us.

The aboriginal Americans wrung reluctant admiration from the newcomers. We can see that if they had been armed as we were armed, if America had been as full of Indians as Europe of Europeans, we could have done no more than establish a beach head on the Atlantic coast. The Indians were the inventors of what we now call commando fighting; we complained of its treachery, and it is indeed a terrible thing to be at war with savage people. But it is a terrible thing, too, for untaught savages to be up against civilized warfare. The Indians defending their homes against men with firearms were like modern infantry without tanks and planes. By the time the Indians had guns and horses, as they did in the Far West when we got there, we had cannon and a regular army, with a line of forts which could be gradually pushed forward. Even so, it was probably our epidemics and our fire-water that demoralized the tribes and broke their spirits. Yet it's famous that with a band of thirty-eight men, and eight boys, Geronimo the Apache terrorized the Southwest and had five thousand army cavalrymen galloping around the desert in circles after him. Today 'Geronimo!' is the exultant war-cry of the American paratroopers when they jump.

For today we are all Americans together. As a race question, the Indian problem, that for three hundred years and more was a bitter war, is simply disappearing. Indians are going to the blood banks to give their plasma for American troops, and if there are any whites who would rather die than have it in their veins, they must belong to a dying kind of American. We just don't want a race problem with the Indians any more, and when that happens, the evil cloud that is a race problem vanishes in light. John Randolph had the blood of Pocahontas in his veins; Will Rogers was a good part Indian. We who have no red man's blood in us have to admit, to the man or woman who has, that they've got the older family and are the more American for it.

The day of the American Indian's sorrow, his humiliation and poverty, is ending. His tribe increases; in Montana, for instance, the white population declined two per cent in the last decade, whereas the Indian increased thirty-five per cent. It's the same wherever there are Indians in any number; it's probable that a century from now the red men will be more numerous and more powerful than they were in 1491.

But though they are multiplying, they are dying too, these days, and for just what they always died for — the land of the free and the home of the brave. Not one single brave on the Jicarilla Apache reservation asked for draft deferment. Their courage is undiminished by civilization. The boldest man his superiors ever saw, they say, was Private Lester Reymus, a full-blood Piute, who beheld a plane crash amid gas tanks at Spartanburg, South Carolina; while it became a torch of fire, and gasoline cans were exploding all around it, this son of our ancient enemies dashed through the flames, into their very heart, and extricated the pilot. The first Indian to die in this war was killed at Pearl Harbor on December 7; his name was Henry Nolatubby, a Chilocco Indian from Oklahoma. A fellow Indian that Sunday morning, Corporal Hermann Boyd, from Washington State, was wounded, but as fast as his blood flowed, he kept blazing away at Jap planes, and won the Order of the Purple Heart for it.

There are plenty of white men as brave as that, of course, but there are services an Indian can perform for his country which white men cannot do. For example, we are up against the fact that thousands of Japanese soldiers, to say nothing of Germans, speak perfect English, indeed, know idiomatic American; consequently our communications can be tapped, and even interlined with misleading statements and commands; even the knottiest code may be deciphered by experts on the other side. But it's a baffled enemy who hears two red men exchanging orders over the field telephones in their native syllables. Navajos are especially used for this work because there are more of their tribe in the armed services than of any other. As their original tongue did not include many technical terms of modern warfare, they have agreed upon jabberwocky equivalents which would have astonished their ancestors.

The Indian soldier is tough. He has lived outdoors all his life, and lived by his senses; he is a natural Ranger. He is wary as a fox, and as silent; he is savage as an injured bear. You may smile, if you want to, when you hear that the Nez Percés at Lapwai have dug up the hatchet, that the Flatheads are on the warpath, and that for the first time in fifty-two years the Sioux have danced a war dance; led by old One Bull, ninety-seven years old, his body still scarred where he gashed himself before going out to fight Custer on the Little Bighorn, two thousand Sioux braves marched off to present themselves before the army recruiting officers. These things are not funny to the Axis, nor can they be comprehensible. To an enemy that has battened on race hatred, our handclasp of truce with the American Indian must be a mystery. But everything that made him such a blood-curdling foe makes him a wonderful brother now.

And this time we're not only physically on the same side, but spiritually. For the American Indian does not have to be sold on democracy; he's always had it. There was one fatal weakness in his pre-Columbian life; he spent his best energies fighting other Indians. This time he's out to scalp some tribes that need their hair lifted, and when our red soldiers vowed to do a war dance in Berlin and Tokyo, we understood that it was no figure of speech. They mean it, and we'll see them do it.

The conflict of the red American with the white American was tragic from start to finish; it was tragic in the Greek sense, not pathetic like a preventable accident, but a predestined clash of irreconcilable forces. No one ever spoke for the red man better than Kit: 'He was a brave man, but he barred the wrong passage.' Now there is no passage for him to bar, or for us to bar to him; we have all got through together.

17

Strange Bird Calling

IF MY FRIEND BALDUR OLden could have read thus far, he might well say that I have not got on with what I started; I have hardly explained my country to him, and this I freely admit. I let loose enthusiasms in this book which I have neglected; I was going to tell about Marblehead in our War of 1812, and how its harbor sheltered the frigate *Constitution* and its men were in her rigging and on her decks in battle. I was going to tell about Jefferson's home, Monticello, and how he built it himself, using his worn copy of Euclid and his true inner eye to raise under the soft Virginia sky a style new upon our sod. I've been meaning to write about the town meetings of New England, the core of democratic self-government; Jefferson gave it the ultimate praise when, the people in those meetings having opposed his Embargo Act, he acknowledged, 'I felt the foundations of the government shaken under my feet by the New England townships.' I meant to tell about Haym Salomon, the little Jew broker who, in the darkest hours of the Revolution, found the market for our bills of exchange when there was no market for them, and died impoverished of the consumption got in a British dungeon. And I ought to have got in Washington's noble reply, 'to the Hebrew gentlemen of Charleston, South Carolina,' when they, who knew what oppression is, congratulated him upon his victory at Yorktown.

For the great writers of America, Baldur, have not usually been our poets and novelists, but our statesmen. Foreign students of our young literature have seldom thought of looking in the decisions of the Supreme Court for the highest thoughts expressed in the inevitably right prose. And not even our own professors of English refer to the speeches and letters of Abraham Lincoln as the greatest prose style of our land. The oratory of Daniel Webster, the joshing of Sam Clemens, the sermons of Emerson, these are our literature, and they are our soul.

But I can't get these in for Baldur Olden, and I don't have to bring them to the attention of my friend Heck; they are so much a part of his thought that when he quotes them he doesn't even use quotation marks.

It seems that, after all, I've been taking my own advice — writing a book I wanted to read and couldn't find anywhere. Because what I want to read about these days is courage, our kind. I know that our enemies have courage, but it's either blind or it's perverted, or both. I would rather be the coward I probably am than brave in the wrong way. Moral courage lies in being brave for the right thing, and without moral courage physical bravery is no better than savage.

That's what makes Tom Paine and Thomas Jefferson greater men than those who lead an attack without thinking why. That's why Lincoln emerged as the greatest hero of the Civil War. It is a noble conscience that makes a man's acts heroism.

There are men who have such consciences in every town, in every age; there are so many, many of them right now that I find I can keep to no theme except this one of courage. But when we find one out, we experience a triumph of our own in the discovery, especially when our unexpected hero died thinking himself a failure.

In the pages of his own writing, I have found such a hero of my own. He bears a famous name, but it was not he who made it famous. John Woodhouse Audubon was the son of the great John James. In the years of the gold rush he went west, and what happened to him then he recorded. Also his daughter Maria wrote a memoir of her father, and I will begin my story — which is a true one — with a sentence of hers. 'On the evening of Tuesday, February 18th,' (1862) she writes, 'he was playing on his violin some of the Scotch airs of which he was so fond.'

Let us listen.

As Jane sank her thin, thirteen-year-old fingers into the familiar opening chords, John Woodhouse Audubon took up his bow and tucked the violin under his chin. His seven other children, his wife Caroline, and his widowed mother Lucy composed themselves to listen. Jane, needing but an occasional glance between the candles at the music, kept her adoring eyes sparkling into her father's, her lips parted in eagerness for his first notes that sounded to her like the piping of merry birds. Because she had always been so happy playing it with him, it did not occur to her that *Loch Lomond* was a sad song. No more could she realize that her father was now a sad man.

His wife, his mother, and his three grown daughters, Lucy, Harriet, and Maria, could see tonight that he did not look well. The boys, being younger, were as careless of it as little Florence; they took the familiar strength of character in the rugged, bearded face for strength of body. He cast one glance of loving concern over them all, and the notes of the violin went dancing wistfully all around the firelit parlor, that seemed more crowded than it was for the billow of crinolines.

The high road and the low road, John Audubon was thinking — the way of those above the ground, the journey of those beneath it! Never in the history of his beloved country had so many at once been taking the low road. And so many more to set out upon it, he saw, before there would be peace between the brothers! Before the wild geese would fly up the Mississippi undisturbed by the gunboats, and the swamp angels sing priestly vespers in the woods where now the short-nosed mortars bellowed the siege of Charleston. It was a small matter, in a cloven nation, that the war had ruined him. But it had once been easier to be confident, in dreadful times more personally imminent than these. For then he had been young, and his future was not then behind him.

Where we twa ha' spent sae mony happy days — sang the bow upon the strings. He did not know that his brown eyes were faithfully smiling into the little girl's.

He had been half Jane's age when he first realized the world did not understand that his father was the kindest and greatest of men. That was on the day when the sheriff of Henderson had come and stripped the Audubon house, in the name of the law of the Commonwealth of Kentucky. John and his older brother Victor, standing pressed against the log walls as the furniture was carried out, scanned their parents' faces to see what they were to think of this. And to their amazement they read that, in some way for which they had never been prepared, the sheriff had the cold rights of it. But when that terrifying official opened the portfolio of John James Audubon's bird paintings, and threw them back as not worth taking, little John knew that the sheriff was wrong nevertheless.

For he knew too that his father followed a call that other people could not hear. Young John used to think it was just the birds of Kentucky's woods, for his father would leave the mill any time that he heard a new whistle. But John Woodhouse Audubon, in his thirty-seventh year, had himself heard the strange bird calling.

It had begun right here, on the bonny, bonny banks of the Hudson, when he had told his mother of his plans for the expedition, and she had smiled slowly, as though it were all an old story to her.

'Of course you must go,' she had readily said. 'You've been looking west for years now.'

'Caroline thinks,' he remarked, 'I may well repair our fortunes, in the gold fields. The Lord knows they need it.'

Lucy smiled again, a little dryly. 'It's what your father always believed when he started out. But it was never the reason he went.'

It hadn't been his son's reason, either. He wanted to complete the mighty lifework of John James Audubon — to see and hear, to know and paint all the birds of the American continent. The genius-woodsman had grown old too early to have known the Western birds in the life. He never crossed the Rockies, never even glimpsed their snow caps; he never watched water ouzels in the white clattering torrents; saw condors soaring on the rivers of the air, nor heard the cascading rapture of the canyon wren. Old eagle of a man, with filming eyes, John James's wings were folded, as his son prepared to set forth. In the eyrie above the Hudson, looking westward, he lived still, but in a remote world of his own. When John bent to kiss him good-bye, he closed his hand with an unexpected strength upon his son's, detaining him. For a long moment, however, it appeared that the clouded brain had lost what it wanted to give. Gently young John began to loosen his fingers, when his father spoke, in a whisper. 'Listen!' he said. And then he was silent, and soon his son departed.

The shore of Texas was no more than first revealed to John Woodhouse Audubon when his heart was already a burden in his breast. Leaning upon the rail of the *Globe*, beside his commander Colonel Webb, he watched the coast come clearer, nearer. The Colonel, thumbs in his belt, patted his hips in anticipation. The land smell blew to them, hot, alien, heavy laden, and Webb drew it in expansively. John was staring along the barrier reefs and bars with unsmiling gaze, for on them he perceived strewn wreckage — ships that had come to this siren shore on ventures no riskier than this one. The farther stranded hulks were ghostly, half-hidden in the pall of spume forever flung up by the breakers. Each nearer hulk, John could see, still had a crew — of solemn brown pelicans squatting on the tipped gunwales and slant spars. As this newcomer ship approached, they lifted on cumbersome wing and in a low and heavily flapping file passed above the upturned faces of the men on the *Globe's* deck.

'It's really a short cut we're taking,' the Colonel was telling John, 'even though it looks longer on the map than the Overland and the Santa Fé trails. Starting in March as we have, and crossing the trunk of Mexico, where there are pacified Indians, on a route horses can traverse, a route I know myself, we'll be at the mines ahead of the lot of them. Why, the New York fortune-hunters will still be wallowing seasick around the Horn! The Illinois hayseeds will be leaving their scalps all along the Apache trails! But, on Webb's Mexican cut-off —' He took a last relishing draw on the butt of his cigar and flung it in an exuberant arc over the rail. A laughing gull swooped past it, stooped where it floated, rose in disgust and gave the brave Colonel its cackling mew of derision.

Gold-hunters though they were, these men were bringing gold with them — twenty-seven thousand dollars of it, invested by themselves and their families and friends, to finance the expedition. In New Orleans, they had discovered, it would be impossible to insure this gold across the harbor bar at Brazos, and once you saw the wrecks along the bar, you knew why. It gives us an insight into the Colonel's character to read in John's journal of the expedition that (though Webb fumed and worried continually about the gold, and told everyone how his responsibilities weighed upon him, as leader and the only military man in the expedition,) when it came to putting the hard metal ashore, he left it to his second in command.

So John at the tiller, and two of the men from the Audubon place at the oars of the small boat, took the jingling treasure ashore through a shallow inlet. On the beach the black skimmers stirred as the boat came near; they opened sarcastic beaks; they rose like a dark curtain blown by some draft — a curtain that swirled before the eyes, hiding all for a moment, then parted, to show raw Brazos squattering on its sands, slumbering, John thought, under that shimmer of precocious heat like a man in a fever dream.

At Brazos, the Colonel with the men under him tarried for nothing, not gold nor rest nor responsibility. John and Jim Clement and Biddle Boggs were left to load the gold on horses and start inland to join the others at Brownsville. They set forth from the desolate sun-bitten settlement hungry and parched with thirst, for they had not touched food nor drink in Brazos. As they rode out onto the coastal savannas, a rumored dread clung to them like an odor. Or, what is harder to escape, the memory of an odor. The skin could not seem to get clean of it. Clem was the first to give it the body of words.

'Maybe it's not what they claim, Mister John,' he suggested, over the thudding hoofbeats.

'It might be that it was real bad last week, Mister John, and all over by now,' said Boggs.

'Don't think about it, Mister John,' begged Clem, with a glance at the grave young face. 'I don't want to think about it, that's a fact,' he pleaded.

'Then let's not talk about it,' John answered him, with his rare gay smile of reassurance.

Clem and Biddle grinned a little ruefully, and pushed their hats back to mop their brows. Shade was only a distant promise, like a mirage, that would not be kept; it lay out of reach under the far-off dreamy *resacas*, the high groves of hackberry and ebony trees that never drew nearer but drifted in green atolls far to the north and south.

Over the tripled hoofbeats sounded the shaken gold they convoyed. The upland plovers, as the horsemen came, rose through the dead air whistling sweetly as a cool wind, and settled again behind them in peaceful hundreds. They do not drag chains of gold across the continent, John thought, nor do they scratch for more. The plovers fly from the pampas to the prairies, and are not afraid. For there is no earth-borne taint upon them. And he too shivered, though he had never known such consuming heat as this on the road to Brownsville. And still on the boat up the Rio Grande, to the Mexican side opposite Fort Ringgold, the heat held. There the expedition was to encamp for four days, while the Colonel traded for horses. Four days — the incubation period for Asiatic cholera.

The old horror was haunting his feverish blood as he laid his bow on the piano. Jane turned the page that ended *Loch Lomond*. 'Please, Father, mayn't we do next that long one about the shipwreck?'

'*The Ballad of Sir Patrick Spens?* By all means,' he said, with his mind still running on the dread that had today so strangely revived in him. What it was born of he did not know, but it filled him, body and brain.

Jane plunged with young vigor into the rhythm; well taught by the metronome, she marched ahead with her chords. I have never been so short of breath, thought her father, fiddling hard to keep abreast of her, and he besought her ruefully with his eyes. But she was reading the words between the bars of music:

> They hoisted their sails on Monenday morn
> Wi' a' the speed they may —

And her father saw the canvas tents going up again, under that long-ago Texas sun. By the Colonel's orders, the little hot white roofs ran in rigid streets down through bogs, up into the cat's-claw and thorny mesquite and out upon the burning sands. The flag had been raised before the Colonel's tent, and promptly at sundown had been lowered; all night the sentries patrolled the camp. What military discipline could command was under control.

One tent was lamplit. There Doctor Perry was searching out the fluttering pulse in a limp wrist. 'Just a touch of cholera morbus,' he said at last, patting the writhing boy's shoulder. 'That's Latin for schoolboy bellyache, Lambert. Probably drank too much water when you were overheated.' He turned away with a dark face and drew John Audubon out of the tent. 'You'll have to tell his brother,' he murmured, 'what it really is.'

Strange Bird Calling

Toward dawn, the sick boy lay in a stupor, and his brother, huddled on the ground with his head in his arms on Lambert's bed, had fallen into the sleep of exhaustion. Audubon stepped out of the tent to draw a breath. The rows of pale canvas were dripping with unlikely dew, and the very ground gave up its own ghosts in curling fumes. It was shortly before sun-up. This is the hour, beside the Rio Grande del Norte, when the chachalaca calls. It is a harsh-voiced fowl, and over and over it proclaimed its monotonous lament. *Tchatch-alack!*

Alack, alack! ran the echo in John Audubon's head. Around him in their helpless sleep lay men who had signed up for this expedition because the son of John James Audubon was going. And at home, awaiting their return, were the people, old friends of the family, who had pressed his hand, their eyes blinded with bright tears. 'I wouldn't send him if you weren't going, John; but you're the son of your father — we all know that.' — 'He's my brother, John, and I know he'll follow you, to the death.' — 'Take care of my boy, Mr. Audubon, he's all I've got in the world.'

Tchatch-alack, crowed the bird in the arid, Mexican waste, *Tchatch-alack!*

As her fingers twinkled over the keys, Jane was singing a soft answer to the violin:

> O lang, lang may the ladies sit
> Wi' their fans into their hand,
> Before they see Sir Patrick Spens
> Come sailing to the land!

Long, long, thought her father, fiddling wearily — how long, O Lord, were those hours. By mid-morning the sky was a brassy bowl wherein the buzzards hovered, high but persistent, passing over the camp like dread across the heart. Somewhere in the mesquite the Inca dove perched, insisting through the hours upon its two sole notes: *No hope. No hope.* Just after noon Lambert was black in the face and dead.

All the hushed camp knew now. They said, 'Just one case.' 'Poor Lambert,' they said, 'he never was up to this trip.' 'A frail boy, anyway.' And they buried him over on the American side. The rich man who owned that land gave a piece of it for the grave, but he wouldn't come near. He had a Mexican wife, who shuddered and stayed away too, but her father, called Don Francisco, came riding out from the ranch, a solitary old figure of dignified compassion. Among Webb's men he stood, lean and erect and gallant with his barbed silvery beard and mustachios, and while Audubon read the service for the dead, Don Francisco crossed himself devoutly. A heretic and lonely burial, he must have thought this; he would sanctify it as he could.

It was John who struck the little canvas house of death. He carried Lambert's clothes and bedding to a pile — even Lambert's brother did not help — and set them afire. He filled in with earth the poisonous trench behind the tent; he burned the lattice of sticks and leaves he had made that morning to keep the sun off the cloth roof while Lambert lived. The fire licked and crackled, pale in the blast of afternoon sunshine. Even the Inca dove now kept a silence like convinced despair.

One of the men who had come along from the Audubon place 'to look after Mister John' was a young giant they called Ham Boden. He was the next to be stricken.

'Where does it hurt, Ham?' tenderly John asked, bending over him.

Ham looked straight back. 'My wife and children hurt, Mr. John.'

He could see Ham's eyes still, as he had said that.

> And there lies gude Sir Patrick Spens
> Wi' the Scots lords at his feet.

Having dragged her father through the whole twenty-two stanzas, Jane clapped her hands in applause of so thorough a tragedy as this they had celebrated. 'Now what about *Flow Gently?*'

'But if your father's tired,' put in Caroline anxiously.

They were all looking at him, he felt, with a concern he must not let them suffer. He was past fatigue now, borne up by the intensity of a sense of life.

'Tired?' he answered, smiling back at them. 'With all of you there to listen to us?' My wife and children! A man is never tired of life, he thought, when it has been so good to him, who is so unworthy. Old Lucy was watching him with a sharp scrutiny of her dark eyes, and he begged, like a boy again, '*Sweet Afton* is one of my favorites, Mother.' For it meant to him Maria, his first wife and truest love.

> Flow gently, sweet Afton, among thy green braes;
> Flow gently, I'll sing thee a song in thy praise;
> My Mary's asleep by thy murmuring stream —

His eyes as he played were on Harriet and young Lucy, hers of all his children. She had been young as Harriet now when she died — sixteen when he first saw her, on the stairs of that Charleston house to which he had come with his father. His fiddle in one hand, his paint box in the other, he had stood staring up at Maria, lost to her in that moment. And she had come running down the stairs with that quick warmth that was never to fail him, to greet her father's dearest friend and offer the Bachman hospitality.

> Thou stock-dove whose echo resounds through the glen —

But not that cloying dove of the Old World, for Maria. It was the mourning dove that always called to him with her voice. Down there on the delta of the Rio Grande there had been many doves, the white-winged, that gave a deep guttural note, and another with a gruff coo almost like an owl's hoot, and the unfamiliar Mexican ground dove. He had thought wearily, hearing them, knowing the sick men around him were dying and that others walking hale and well would sicken, that nothing so presses unhappiness in upon the heart as the calling of alien birds. That they are not known to a man makes them sound unfeeling, and if there is beauty in their notes it is beauty without heart for you. So, when he heard the one bird there in Texas that he loved, it seemed to have a mind to him. *Ah!* came the first indrawn and rapturous breath, followed by the three cool notes, *coo — coo — coo!* And Maria was beside him, almost the rustle of her gown, surely the strength of their love giving his sick heart courage.

He leaned against the piano, letting little Jane play the rest of the melody in a solo. There was upon him some strange compulsion tonight to live over to the end that adventure in Texas which had been the climax and the failure of all his hopes. So he sorted out those last events of it now in his mind. How the Colonel himself had deserted, alleging in a letter sent his second, after his own departure, that he went to get horses from the Mexicans. How John had been counseled to take the gold to the American side and there deposit it.

'We're striking camp,' ordered John, straightening his shoulders under the burden. 'Burn everything that has been touched. In the morning put the sick in wagons, and the poor lads in their coffins into another, and bring them over the Rio Grande. I'll go ahead into town to make ready.'

The Armstrong Hotel, as Audubon dismounted at two in the morning, was still a blaze of lights. There was cholera in Rio Grande City too, but no halt in the fun at Armstrong's. Out of the windows blew gusts of drunken laughter and breaking glass, and the long rumbling thunder followed by a crash and yells of triumph, that is nothing but a bowling alley. The place was crowded with a bar and drinking tables, and around other tables, where monte and faro were going full tilt, pressed prairie boys with their big hats on the backs of their heads, halfbreed women, Mexicans draped in serapes, beaver-hatted adventurers, scum of New Orleans and Natchez-Under-the-Hill, affecting the manners of rice-planting gentry.

John saw the gold safely into the hotel's strong box, then stumbled up to fall on his bed in the haunted sleep that follows disaster. Into his face laughed the faces of boys he had loved who were now suddenly dead — Ham Boden, Bill Harrison,

Whittlesey, Liscomb, and bonny young Howard Bakewell, his own mother's favorite nephew. Below, the fatalists kept up their mad rejoicing, the thunderous bowls knocking down pins as the cholera knocks men down.

His head thudded, his bow hand dropped tiredly to his side; while Jane pranced on with the melody, John Audubon knew now that sickness was upon him. He burned with fever. The long-past events he was pursuing ran faster in his mind. How in the morning the gold had been gone from the safe, and no one could be found to admit it had ever been there. Death and disorder were in this place, and thieves conspired easily among them. Then the thief was caught and, under threat of lynching, led John and his men to the spot on the lonely prairie where in the night he had buried the gold. And the gold was gone.

John drew a hard breath as little Jane finished. 'Let's do *Lord Randall*, Janie,' he urged. 'All the old songs have something to say to me tonight.'

There was a burden upon him as heavy as the gold had weighed; he felt a dread like that the wagons brought, rumbling into town with the sick and dying; he tried to escape from it, into the music, and could not. He was standing here by Jane's piano, and yet he was standing, too, over those open graves of boys dead with cholera, reading aloud the burial service: 'Man that is born of woman hath but a short time to live —' The deep chords of it sounded in his mind under the song's melody,

— make my bed soon,
For I'm sick to the heart, and I fain wad lie doon.

With just this dark prescience the cholera had struck him. He could remember how the gold had seemed to be pouring over him in a hard, heartless stream, crushing him with the weight of responsibility for it, gold that he did not want, gold that dazzled men and killed them off like flies. He must have been delirious a long time. His head, he remembered, only began to clear when old Don Francisco was standing in his tent, telling him that the gold was safe. 'I see thees men bury your money in the night, in the *resaca*. Was I not once *gerifa* here? So when they go away, I deeg it up, señor. I keep it safe for you.'

So the weight lifted from his body, and the darkness passed from his mind. A long time John lay still, after the old man went, looking at the late sunlight through the open tent flaps. He was going to get well, he knew now. They had told him that the cholera was passing. By some coincidence, Colonel Webb had returned to take command. And was turning the party back, accepting defeat, taking the easy way out.

The camp was very silent, John thought. The men who had come in to visit him had been silent too, near to broken. They had been led here to Texas confidently, and they themselves had been faithful. They were faithful still, but bewildered, betrayed. What was left for them but, leaderless, to follow the retreat of their former leader?

None of the birds of Texas were singing at this hour. But John began to listen, as his father had bade him. Far, far away, as far as the greenwood bridal that had borne him, came the strange voice calling. It is always from beyond that it whistles, calling a man to take the hard way, to do the thing that perhaps cannot be done, to get through somehow — yes, and to get the others through, those others who look to him. Now the dusk was falling over the camp. The men, lingering in groups, looked up and stared as he came wavering out of his tent. 'Boys,' he called clearly to them all, 'I'm not giving up. I'm not going back. Who will go on with me?'

'Play *Onward Christian Soldiers*, Janey,' her father said feverishly. 'Play it and sing it, all of you! For me.'

He leaned against the piano, hearing through the martial hymn the shouts of the men who acclaimed him. 'On with

Audubon! John Audubon to lead us!' But it was his family singing; *Marching as to war!* A tragic exhilaration seized him. He had got them through, over desert and wilderness to promised California.

And none of them struck gold, none of them became rich. Instead, they became carpenter, lawyer, cook, doctor, engineer, teacher; each found his place in the new land that needed them. They found no gold. They brought their gold with them, a deep vein of the best human metal, in every man.

So it was over; under Jane's fingers the last chord echoed through the room. He was very tired; he must get to bed. He thought that the birds he had followed were flying past his blurred vision. Pass softly, he thought, as he laid his violin on the piano, and stepped away over the carpet — pass softly where the lark is building hidden on the sod; be quick of eye for the little skull that once held wary eyes and hungry palate. The half of a robin's egg, lying empty in the grass — be tender of it, and of the grass itself you walk upon. '"In the morning it is green;"' John Audubon was murmuring as he left the room, '"and groweth up: but in the evening it is cut down, dried up, and withered."' The door closed quietly upon him.

They say that as he sank into his final delirium that night he talked constantly of the end of his Texas venture. The bitterness of what he thought his great failure came from between his lips, released at last from the depth where he had hidden it. He spoke of the collections he had made that were lost in shipwreck around the Horn, of his drawings that were scattered on the Gila desert, forsaken because the sick men had demanded his attention instead. He had never been able to complete his father's giant task. He was no giant himself, like the great John James. He had only been faithful, and failed.

Failed, John?

Ninety-eight men had set forth, self-confident, the glint of riches in their eyes. One carried the sick in his arms to their beds, comforted their grief, closed their eyes, and read the word of God above them. One cleansed what others would not touch, shouldered what others would not carry, led on when others turned back. To do so much that is so hard, as John Woodhouse Audubon did it, one must hear a clear call. True that he was no genius, like his father. But the strange bird calls to all of us who will listen.

18

'The Great and Durable Question'

FROM THE FIRST, THE settlers in this new-found land saw that autumn was our crowning season. So they gave a new name to it — the name of fall. To English ears, I'm told, this Americanism sounds unpoetic, almost illiterate. To our ancestors the fall of the leaves, in the close-pressing menace of the primeval forest, meant a long view through the woods, where the Indian could no longer ambush, and the leaping buck and strutting wild turkey were clear on the sights of the rifle at last. So they called it fall, let Oxford sigh as it might, and they learned that fall was the time of all times for pressing westward, in those annual growth rings by which our country expanded. For the flood waters of spring were down, and there was dry ground for the creaking wheels of the wagons. The summer fevers and flies were gone, and the winter cold and hunger not yet come. The game was fat and plenty, and the pawpaw and persimmon were ripe and plashy on the stem. And it seemed to the pioneers that the autumn winds, out of the west, blew them the tang of destiny. So they rode, or walked, upwind under the tapestries of autumn, and the purple vervain bowed beneath their wheels and the black walnuts rained sweet kernels at their feet.

Now this national feeling that autumn belongs to America is not just a provincial fancy. If there is one thing on which

European observers are agreed to yield the honors to a country which they view askance in so many things, it is the way that Nature does up autumn on the North American continent. Kipling and Lord Bryce have paid their tribute. Audubon gloried in the American fall. Even from Mrs. Trollope, the harshest critic we ever had, not excepting Dickens, our fall wrung reluctant admiration:

> Our autumn walks were delightful.... I never saw so many autumn flowers as grow in the woods and sheep-walks of Maryland; a second spring seemed to clothe the fields.... The trees took a coloring which in richness, brilliance, and variety, exceeds all description. I think it is the maple or sugar-tree that first sprinkles the forest with rich crimson; the beech follows, with all its harmony of golden tints, from pale yellow up to brightest orange. The dogwood gives almost the purple color of the mulberry; the chestnut softens all with its frequent mass of brown..... The colors are in reality extremely brilliant, but the medium through which they are seen increases the effect surprisingly. Of all the points in which America has the advantage of England, the one I felt most sensibly was the clearness and the brightness of the atmosphere. By day and by night this exquisite purity of air gives tenfold beauty to every object.

But the good lady was not able to pour the mead of praise for anything over here without a drop of wormwood in it. She finds that the senseless uproar of the autumn woods and fields in America, with all its locusts, grasshoppers, katydids, and crickets, reminds her of the hurly-burly of our fall election campaigns:

> Even in retirement we were not beyond the reach of the election fever, which is constantly raging through the land. Had America every attraction under heaven that Nature and social enjoyment can offer, this electioneering madness would make me fly it in disgust.

But to an American the fall elections, held in a season of sharpened atmosphere, are a time of national self-examination. We examine not only our candidates and their parties and platforms. We look into ourselves, and we ask what America stands for? We remember that it is not an old and static nationalism, but an experiment in human nature. Its past is so recent that we feel as though we could actually turn to Webster or Clay, the two Wilsons — James and Woodrow — to Jackson or to John Adams, and say, what would you have us do, in these circumstances? And you, Long Tom? You, Abraham Lincoln?

His voice still can be heard, over the soft rustle of the falling hickory leaves. For it was in the autumn of 1858 that Lincoln went on record to the nation, and his words still carry a living challenge. At that time all men had come to perceive that there was a deep rift in the Union. The whole country centered attention on the Lincoln-Douglas debates. In Illinois, town and hamlet and farm came gathering to hear the crucial argument. Over the sunburnt prairie the buggy wheels came rolling, where the asters smoked and ironweed and goldenrod smouldered; the burr oak and shagbark dropped slow big dry leaves in the groves where the buggies were tethered. For in these small Illinois towns there were no audience halls large enough to hold so large a question, so great a crowd as those that came to hear threshed out the subject of slavery in the Union.

The two speakers had to begin almost every debate by begging the audience to remain profoundly quiet so that their voices might be heard to the last ring of buggies and wagons where the horses cropped the bluegrass and redtop and the children napped. But once the issues were before the audience, there was no need to ask for quiet. A hush like death, we are told, prevailed. For every listener soon understood that the life of the Union was approaching crisis, and the meaning of democracy — New World, American democracy — must now be defined and then upheld. Men saw a civil war approaching; for some it could not come fast enough — a surgeon's knife to let out poisoned blood. Others sought to escape it by hiding their faces in their hands, like people who see that their boat is being swept toward disaster. Politically the subject of slavery was a rock to founder on. Conservatives in all parties wanted to flow around this sharp black reef which reared in midchannel of our destiny. But as the ship was swept on toward it, no one in the country, at last, could avoid or avert meeting the question. In the campaign debates before the election for senator from Illinois, in 1858, the smoothest, most powerful and popular standpat politician in the country was brought to bay by the barking voice of a lean hound from the Sangamon River country, whose nose for the real and moral issue could not be confused by any political cross-scents dragged across the trail.

In 1619, at Jamestown, Virginia, John Rolfe, the husband of Pocahontas (who certainly showed no race prejudice) recorded, 'Came in a Dutch man of warre that sold us twenty Negars.' So the African reached our soil one year before the Pilgrims, ancestors of many of the Abolitionists, set foot on Plymouth Rock. Less than twenty years later, so I have read, a Salem speculator ordered built for him, in the shipyards of Marblehead, a vessel with the strange and beautiful name of *Desire*; in this he brought back slaves captured in the jungles of Africa. It was the first American boat to run the infamous Middle Passage — that is, neither the North Atlantic to Europe nor around the Horn or Cape of Good Hope for the spice, silk, and tea trade, but down along the Equator where the Niger and the Congo pour their dark floods into the waters of the world.

So the negro problem was already two hundred years old, that fall of national crisis; it was a problem of race relations, it was an economic problem, and lastly it was a problem of the American democratic revolution. What, men asked, had the signers of the Declaration of Independence, and the framers of the Constitution, intended with respect to the rights of the negro or our rights in him? This last was the most painful question of all, for if there is anything that a politician does not want injected into a campaign, it is a moral issue. When people begin to vote by their consciences, parties crack up; even regulars cannot be held in line; oratory has no charm; established political personalities may go into the discard; the times grow revolutionary. Laws may be disobeyed, and proudly. National tradition is blown from the page of history as if it were dust.

But not lightly. Americans of those days, both North and South, were predominantly religious, in most cases deeply so. They referred their problem to Scripture, and both closed the Good Book, fortified. Both felt themselves to be defenders of the original intention of the founders of the American commonwealth. The tragic fact is that both were. For those founders, our Revolutionary ancestors, were as divided upon slavery, and almost as divided upon the meaning of the American union, as were our Civil War ancestors. Of necessity, they buried the hatchet; we can see them doing it, deliberately and consciously, in the course of the Constitutional Convention. Now the floods had washed the hatchet up. It shone where no one could avoid seeing it, and hands that would reach for it were now stirring.

Not long before the Lincoln-Douglas debates, two pieces of print had struck like lightning. One was a novel, *Uncle Tom's Cabin*, by a square-faced New England widow — a book which as a novel and in play form has commanded more audiences in remote corners of the earth than any other product from an American pen. If a cool modern wonders how our forebears could have been taken in by so much Victorian sentimentality and lamentable taste, let him remember that those readers were Victorian and they had the taste fashionable in their day, as we have in ours. Let him remember that Americans are the most compassionate people in the world, especially about the sorrows of the oppressed who are removed at some little distance from them — the Flatheads, the Zulus, the Belgians under the heel of Wilhelm Hohenzollern, the negroes under the heel of the Belgians in the Congo Free State. Although it is difficult to make Americans hate, it is not hard to make them fighting mad. And *Uncle Tom's Cabin* made North and South both fighting mad.

Into this tense atmosphere came a document, the decision of Justice Taney of the Supreme Court, by which a negro who had escaped to the free-soil territory of Minnesota was sent back in chains to an owner in Missouri. The aged justice's decision was based upon an interpretation of the Constitution, which withheld citizenship from the negro and made him property of which his owner could not be deprived without due process of law. So Dred Scott was returned out of freedom, like a hog that had broken through the fence.

The American people revere the Supreme Court as they will no other body. Senators may be coerced to their knees by popular ridicule; the President is not immune from any sort of verbal attack, but the Supreme Court judges are viewed with awe and almost inviolate from criticism. Their decrees are accepted as though the people were loving children who look up to parents to make wise decisions, whether pleasant or not. The Dred Scott case had those Northerners who opposed slavery baffled; the moral side of their political natures was torn in conflict. Nothing could resolve it except a man who would dare their own fury by standing up and saying that the highest tribunal in the land was utterly mistaken, and that its decision must be reversed.

Even before the great debates were scheduled, Lincoln laid the matter wide open, by a blow to the heart of it with his axeman's arm. In a speech at Springfield he dared, against the advice of his political friends, a most Lincolnian thing: he reached into Scripture and lifted out an eternal truth that lit up all that others wanted only to hide, or hide from. '*A house divided against itself cannot stand.*'

> I believe this government cannot endure half slave and half free.... Either the opponents of slavery will arrest the further spread of it ... or its advocates will push it forward till it shall become alike lawful in all the states.

The Great and Durable Question 243

In the second breath of his speech Lincoln attacked the Dred Scott decision. The keen hound smelled infallibly the moral rat. Unaware of the letters that were one day to come to light, he pieced together the collusion among the justices, Stephen A. Douglas, President Pierce who was just going out, and the standpat, do-nothing, expedient Buchanan who was just coming in. The justices had made up their minds on sectional, political, racial, and economic grounds before ever the case reached them. They held off their decision, though, until the election of Buchanan made it safe to render it, but Douglas, then in the Senate, had known what the decree would be. So he dared to introduce the Nebraska Bill, which in substance opened all the national territory to slavery by local option. This was done under a shield on which was painted the device 'Popular Sovereignty.' Lincoln struck that shield a cracking blow.

> The 'sacred right of self-government' . . . though expressive of the only rightful base of any government, was so perverted in this attempted use of it as to amount to just this: that if any *one* man chose to enslave *another*, no *third* man shall be allowed to object.

Now he struck at a shadow, one that he recognized as dangerous.

> The Nebraska doctrine . . . is to educate and mold . . . public opinion not to care whether slavery is voted down or voted up.

Not to care — that is where men always begin to lose. Don't look now, but the Redcoats are firing on the civilians of Boston Common. It's not our business, but the Japanese soldiery are raping Nanking. Hitler is prodding the Jews to their graves in quicklime, but that's a matter to leave to the 'sacred right of self-government.'

As Lincoln stood that day before the convention of Republicans that had nominated him, he recognized the wide difference between Douglas and himself. He was a newcomer, though he regarded himself as already old. He was self-taught, little traveled, little read beyond the Bible and Shakespeare and Blackstone — wilderness timber seasoned but not polished. His opponent, called 'the Little Giant,' was the greatest figure in the United States Senate since Webster, Clay, and Calhoun. Like Lincoln, he was a lawyer, but he took only big corporation cases. He voted as an avowed friend of big business and, as usually happens with such politicians, the little business men imagined that he was thereby their friend too. His polish positively glittered, and his tour of Europe had been a royal progress, in which he paused to bow kindly to the Czar. He was a Vermonter, by birth, and was fond of alluding to this fact; he chiseled himself out of granite as he described his ancestry. I have never read an admission from him that his first wife was a Southerner who left him a legacy of one hundred and fifty slaves.

Lincoln and Douglas were old friends — as lawyers reckon friendship; they slapped each other on the back on courtroom steps and beat their breasts at one another in front of the jury. They were old rivals, and so far all the monetary and political success had gone to Douglas. Now Lincoln switched from professional comradeship to political tilting:

> They remind us that he is a great man and that the largest of us are very small ones. . . . But 'a living dog is better than a dead lion.' Judge Douglas, if not a dead lion, for this work is at least a caged and toothless one. How can he oppose the advances of slavery? He don't care anything about it. His avowed mission is impressing the 'public heart' to *care nothing about it.*

Douglas hurried back from the East to answer this. His home city of Chicago met him with a monster torchlight procession. Present, but not speaking that night, barely able to squeeze into the crowd, Lincoln heard Douglas utter, from the balcony of his hotel, his studied periods. The lion roared, tossing back his magnificent dark mane; he was effulgent in the torchlight; he snarled at Biblical quotation; talk like

Lincoln's, he said, was just what would bring on war between North and South. But if we would stop talking about slavery, if we wouldn't keep bringing the matter into the light, there would be no occasion to quarrel over it. He, Douglas, was a law-abiding man, a lawyer who bowed reverently to the decisions of the Supreme Court.

> This government of ours is founded on a white basis. It was made by the white man, for the benefit of the white man, to be administered by white men, in such manner as they should determine.... True that a negro, an Indian, or any other man of inferior race ... should be permitted to enjoy ... all the rights, privileges, and immunities which he is capable of exercising consistent with the safety of society.... You may ask me, what are these rights and these privileges? My answer is that each state must decide for itself the nature and extent of these privileges.

> I do not acknowledge that the negro must have civil and political rights everywhere or nowhere. I do not acknowledge that the Chinese must have the same rights in California that we would confer upon him here.... I am in favor of preserving not only the purity of the blood, but the purity of the government from any admixture or amalgamation of inferior races.

Where have we heard this kind of talk since? Racial purity! Master race! We know now what may follow, quite logically, from accepting such concepts. Douglas's web of argument was perfectly logical; it was a web of steel, and there was no way that anyone obeying the political rules of the game could break it. For it is not good politics to tell your constituents that what they consider their inferiors are their equals before God. But the next day, from the same balcony, Lincoln replied (though Douglas, retiring to his mansion on the South Side, did not deign to be present).

> My friend [Douglas] has said to me that I am a poor hand to quote Scripture. I will try it again, however. It is said in one of the admonitions of our Lord, 'As your Father in Heaven is perfect, be ye also perfect.' The Savior, I suppose, did not

> expect that any human creature could be perfect as the Father in Heaven; but ... he set that up as a standard. ... So I say in relation to the principle that all men are created equal, let it be as nearly reached as we can. If we cannot give freedom to every creature, let us do nothing that will impose slavery upon any other creature. ... I leave you, hoping that the lamp of liberty will burn in your bosoms until there shall no longer be a doubt that all men are created equal.

Right in Lincoln's home town of Springfield, in the debated middle counties of the state, neither clearly proslavery like the southern counties nor Abolitionist like the northern ones, Douglas bellowed, so that the deafest old lady on the furthest rim of the crowd could hear:

> The Declaration of Independence, in the words, 'all men are created equal,' was intended to allude only to the people of the United States, to men of European birth or descent, being white men. ... Did they mean to say that the Indian, on this continent, was created equal to the white man, and that he was endowed by the Almighty with inalienable rights? ... But Mr. Lincoln's conscientious scruples on this point govern his actions, and I honor him for following them, although I abhor the doctrine which he preaches. ... I take great pleasure in bearing testimony to the fact that Mr. Lincoln is a kindhearted, amiable, good-natured gentleman. ... He is a worthy gentleman. ... He is a fine lawyer, possesses high ability, and there is no objection to him, except the monstrous revolutionary doctrine with which he is identified and which he conscientiously entertains and is determined to carry out if he gets the power.

The Senator was smart; he was even just. He saw very well, this Transylvanian, that Lincoln's beliefs and words were revolutionary, and he honestly feared them. The Civil War which was so soon to descend upon thirty-five million people — not one of whom recognized himself as responsible for it — was the second shooting stage of the American Revolution. Everybody talks about it as though the South had gone into rebellion against the Federal Government, a rebellion that failed. I have never seen any historian state what looks to me like an obvious truth: that the nineteenth-century North was in revolution against the eighteenth-century South's interpretation of the Constitution — a revolution that succeeded. If the South wishes to maintain that it was defending the concept of democracy and union which was entertained by a majority of the framers of the Constitution, it is probably entitled to that justification. It fought with the high-mindedness of a people religiously and politically alert. It was the gamest fight Americans ever lost and won. The South, indeed, could say and did think that it was just a little more American, in the old sense, than the North which was swiftly filling up with immigrants. A new America — like it more or like it less — was growing inside the old. The first pains of its terrible birth were felt in the convulsions of the Lincoln-Douglas debates, and people who had never before turned their eyes toward remote Illinois looked now with fear and hope upon that clash of spirits. Longfellow, Greeley, Whittier, Chase, they listened and they began to understand that a moral giant had shouldered up above the Little Giant, when he answered Douglas at Springfield:

> I do not understand the Declaration to mean that all men were created equal in all respects. . . . But I suppose that it does mean that all men are equal . . . in their right to 'life, liberty, and the pursuit of happiness.' Certainly the negro is not our equal in color — perhaps not in many other respects; still, in the right to put into his mouth the bread that his own hands have earned, he is the equal of every other man, white or black. In pointing out that more has been given you, you cannot be justified in taking away the little which has been given him. . . . If God gave him but little, that little let him enjoy.

At Ottawa, under a corn-weather sun, twelve thousand men of Illinois and their bonneted women listened for three hours while the two titans hurled rocks of logic and bolts of lawyer lightning at each other. There was something naked about Lincoln on that day; there was something sorrowful and premonitory as he, a son of Kentucky, a grandson of Virginia, lifted his voice to say:

> I have no prejudice against the Southern people. They are just what we would be in their situation. If slavery did not now exist among them, they would not introduce it. If it did now exist among us, we should not instantly give it up. . . . When Southern people tell us that they are no more responsible for the origin of slavery than we, I acknowledge the fact. . . . It does seem to me that systems of gradual emancipation might be adopted; but for their tardiness in this, I will not undertake to judge our brethren of the South.

Now the two men went together to Freeport. It's a good town; I know that town; I know the editor of the paper there, and his wife. I've been to a Fourth of July picnic at Freeport, and I've driven out from it with the old editor, father of the present one, in a surrey with a fringed top, to see the place, a little way out on the prairie, where Jane Addams was born. In lilac time the town's all loveliness; in summer you can hear, of a hot evening, what the children are practicing on their pianos, up and down the streets. It's pretty cold in winter, but when the sleet bends the telephone lines down in great glittering loops, and the people who went to grand opera in Chicago last night don't get home till sunrise is making rosy crystals of the icy trees, everybody laughs, and they all call each other up to ask if their friends are out of groceries or milk; and, if the car won't start, a neighbor will take your children to school.

In Freeport fifteen thousand people stood in a light drizzle to hear the two lawyers put each other on the stand. For this was electioneering, avowedly, but Freeport would not be shaken from its grip upon the issues behind the election. Never was Douglas so heckled. 'I have seen your mobs before,' he shouted, 'and defy your wrath.' Lincoln talked boldly enough up here, sneered Douglas, but he would drag the 'Tall Sucker' down to Egypt — to southern Illinois populated from the South, wedged between the slave states of

Missouri and Kentucky. 'Why,' Lincoln smiled slowly and broadly to the audience at Jonesboro, 'way down in Egypt land, 'I know this people better than he does. I was raised just a little east of here. I am a part of this people.'

That was in mid-September — the time, in Illinois, when the crows call across a wide, warm stillness, when the goldenrod is bobbing beneath a freight of restless bees all under the oaks and the hickories. In the fields the corn is shocked, and the field mice rustle through it; the farm children go out to turn the pumpkin's colder cheek to the sun. That sun was hot when the two giants wrestled in oratory at Charleston, in the center of the state; the sweat-dewed faces of the country crowd were streaked with the dust raised by the processions bearing banners for Lincoln, for Douglas, by the marching bands and the white-gowned girls. But when October broke, and they spoke in Galesburg, the weather broke too; a breath had come tingling, sparkling down from the northwoods, and now it pulled awry the women's best bonnets and flapped the long coat of the tall man talking on the platform, who had forgotten himself in his words.

Six days later came the debate at Quincy, on the Mississippi; the scribbling pencils of the reporters taking it down in that new-fangled thing, shorthand, sent the words, as before, to speed over all the land. Up in the woods of Minnesota, where Dred Scott had not been free, the free Indians were gathering in their wild rice. In Missouri, where Scott was property, the persimmons fell and the lean hogs rooted for them. Chill winds were sweeping through the high-ceiled rooms of the Saratoga hotels, and the New Yorkers and South Carolinians were having a last drink in the bars together, enemy friends who shook out their newspapers and read of the final debates out there in Illinois at Quincy and Alton, with noddings and shakings. These wiseacres knew how the election would turn out. Lincoln had spent a thousand dollars on the campaign — enough to flatten a small-time lawyer. Douglas had borrowed some sixty thousand dollars; that meant as much to a big lawyer as a thousand to a small one. It meant, too, that the Senator could hardly refuse what his backers might wish him to do — Tammany, railroads, newspapers, bankers, investors. Yes, it was all in the bag. The season was over, and their wives could pack their furbelows, their hoops and bonnets, and start home.

As for the context of the debates, these wise gentlemen had some scorn for both candidates. Lincoln was a fool to get himself mixed up with lunatic reformers — for Douglas had plastered him with the name of Abolitionist, hard as Lincoln fought it. But Douglas was far from satisfying the strongest political thinking in the South. He wasn't advocating secession, and it seemed to Southern leaders like Rhett and Yancey that every minute that the South remained in this riffraff Union she was in worse danger of being defenselessly overwhelmed. So let them chew the rag, out there between the corn rows; let the Suckers listen. Sucker money, sucker votes, simpletons trying to piece out reason, in a crossroads political show! Going to the polls, as November opened, to vote for the dead lion or the living dog.

And of course it all turned out just as they knew it would, in the wards of New York and Charleston. The sixty-thousand-dollar man beat the one-thousand-dollar man. Whose eyes would that widen? The voters played safe, the majority at least; they returned to office a man who, they knew, would get them new postoffices and postmasterships, a man who would keep them out of war, so they liked to believe, and run business as usual. The rooms of Senator Douglas blazed with lights as his congratulators poured into his reception to drink up his whiskies and pump his hand. He didn't exactly object, and he was smart as always; he congratulated the voters. It's always said, at a time like that, that you can rely on the sound good sense of the American people when they go to the polls.

The first snow began to drop, pure and spinning from a gray-goose sky, through the woods of Minnesota. Nobody who was anybody was left in Saratoga, where the American patriots once had rounded up Burgoyne's army and forced it to surrender. In the hotels the chandeliers were tied up in bags, and on the deep verandas, bare of rockers now, the leaves swept whispering along. In Charleston, South Carolina, the families were coming back from Virginia Springs and Flat Rock, rolling up in their carriages to the grille gates; the shutters were flung open and the old mahogany dusted; the mirrors gave back again white features and black, smiling at each other. It was one of the self-deceptions of the slave-owning families that they never noticed how they made their house servants members of the family, giving and taking from them Christian love, but their field servants they might not even know by name and left to the mercy of white men whom they themselves despised.

The country forgot Illinois again; Illinois went on with its business. The farmers had gathered in their corn by now. Lincoln was left like a chill cricket in the stubble. Of the debating that was over, he said:

> It gave me a hearing on the great and durable question of the age which I could have had in no other way; and though I now sink out of view and shall be forgotten, I believe I have made some marks which will tell for the cause of civil liberty long after I am gone.

There is no one left alive who can remember the Lincoln-Douglas debates. But every one of us has debates within himself to remember. There is nobody who is free from twinges, at least, of race prejudice, no one guiltless of assumptions of superiority, of a desire, however momentary, to put some wall or some distance between himself and those racially different from him. We all pour scorn, of course, on the other fellow's bigotry about this matter; it is absurd of him, we say, to see danger in, or feel aversion to, that race or this other. Only our own secret prejudices do we cherish as a virtue. We call them mere common sense, and, if the drums are beating loud enough that year, we call them Americanism.

Yes, we recognize these debates within ourselves. For myself, I recall pictures that illuminated them. I remember the negro as I found him in the Bluegrass. In those luxury spots where fat white columns promise you the best of food inside, the best of service, he warms the complacent heart. He offers you incomparable juleps, fried chicken, corn pudding, cozening you to let him bring you further comforts, his voice soft, supplicating, deferential. He is as pleased with your praise as a dog at a pat on the head. Or you enjoy seeing him standing about on street corners, loose-jointed, tatterdemalion, looking worthless and picturesque.

I remember, too, the convoy of army trucks we passed there near Lexington, manned by negro troops. These men stood straight — brown, lighter brown, black, ebony black, all equalized by khaki. They looked you straight, out of unsmiling faces, as good as you — good enough to die for you.

And I remember the young people I was asked to talk to, here in my town, about the promise of American democracy. I remember how proudly straight they too stood, and how heartily they sang, 'Land where my fathers died.' It made me smile, because their eyes were almond and their fathers had come from Japan. In introducing me, my fellow American citizen Tom Hiroshima said that I was friendly toward the American Japanese and, he added with a wistful twinkle around the four walls, 'We're needing friends just now.' Some laughed at that, and some looked grave. The date was the 5th of December, 1941.

On Sunday, December 7, I called up the young editor of our paper and said, 'Charles, I want time on your radio to talk about our Japanese and I haven't got any money to pay for it.' And he let me speak. I said then, and I say now, that these people in my town were innocent of the crimes of the Tokyo Government. I said that to turn this into a race war was just what Tokyo, and Hitler too, were trying to do. Any American who may be tempted to toy even carelessly with race prejudice had better look well at the bloodstains on it, and shudder away. For that implement of disunion is a planted weapon, and those who go about urging it upon us are themselves tools of the enemy.

The little Buddhist temple wherein I spoke to the Japanese-American Citizens' League has its doors sealed now. The sukiyaki restaurant, and the grocery that used to have rice cakes and teapots in the window, are closed and empty, like all the buildings on that block opposite the postoffice. I feel a sense of desolation when I walk through the Japanese quarter, so-called — it was never anything more than a few houses and stores in among the American Chinese. When our Japanese neighbors had to leave us, all the ministers of this California town put their signatures to a letter of loving farewell. And what the Japanese felt, at their best, was best said by my own old gardener, Yoneda, when we shook hands in good-bye. 'Wherever they send me,' he said with his sad pride, 'it will still be America.'

Will it? Will it be America still for those people, when the war between Japan and ourselves is over? Shall we, through the bloodshed and the grief and the resentment, remember what Abraham Lincoln said, in a little Illinois town?

> What constitutes the bulwark of our liberty and independence? It is not our frowning battlements, our bristling seacoasts, the guns of our war steamers, or the strength of our gallant army. These are not our reliance against a resumption of tyranny in our land. All of them may be turned against our liberties without making us stronger or weaker for the struggle.
>
> Our reliance is in the love of liberty which God has planted in our bosoms. Our defence is in the preservation of liberty as the heritage of *all men, in all lands everywhere.*

The italics are Lincoln's. He was so tall he could see over the heads, and over the corn, and over the years, to our time.

19

Soldiers in the Streets

WE HAD AN ELECTION of our own, here in the Santa Barbara district, some months back, to send a man to Congress. Perhaps because I helped a little, I had for the first time the sense that my candidate, if elected, would really represent this town, our people, and — least important — myself. He was one of us, all right, a teacher in the State College here, a man I'd talked with many a time. I knew his views and he knew mine, and they were just about the same.

His rival was a good man too, I suppose. People said he'd surely get elected because he was a practical business man and he had a mysterious and dreaded thing called 'the machine' behind him, whereas our man was a political dark horse, and, worse, a professor. There were some joint debates between the candidates, and the issue turned — unfortunately for the other fellow — upon foreign policy, the peace to come, and the world to be made after the war. The honorable opponent here complained bitterly. Foreign affairs weren't his line; and George (our man) knew it, whereas George taught history and economics and such, and had it all on his tongue. George's opponent fervently assured the electors that though he might not know much about the theory of international politics, he would get the voters what they wanted, if they sent him to Congress.

Said our George, in effect: If you elect me to the House of Representatives I will put humanity first, America second, California third, Santa Barbara fourth.

We sent him to the House.

I wonder how often he has time, back there in wartime Washington, to remember the town he comes from. Does he ever hear in his head the soft clangor of the Mission bells, coming regularly like the pulsing of an old heart? Or the mockingbirds in the gardens behind the high green hedges, calling on every fine day and every moonlight night, 'Beauty, beauty, beauty! See it, see it, see it! Beauty, whew!'

That's our civic motto, all right. Father Serra saw beauty when he picked this spot, and Father Lasuén created more of it when he built the Queen of the Missions. The old Spanish families — still living, some of them, in the first adobes that were raised upon the little sloping plain between the mountains and the beach — must have settled here because they found it fair; it is hard to see why else they would have stopped here where there was no harbor and no river. But here they planted their olives and oranges, and here, after them, came the Americans. The first of us recorded that nowhere else on earth had the art of sweetly doing nothing been raised to such enjoyable perfection.

In a general sort of a way, the town boomed on that principle. Almost everybody was here because he found life pleasanter in this spot than in any other he could imagine arriving at. Most of us adults were not born here; we came together voluntarily, and, having found a good thing, we met each other on the street with smiles of mutual congratulation which the years did not wear off. Beauty is a cash crop around here, and, beside all the God-given brand, the citizens have done their best to create it. It's the prettiest little city I ever saw in America; it has the riches of civilization upon a jewel-box scale, but it is full of Nature too. The trees elbow the gardens for the sunlight, and as soon as the rush and the bumbling toot of the trains subside, you hear the mockers again. And over everything washes the breath of the Pacific, spring and fall. All summer long you hear the swish of children's roller skates and the bubbling of the wren-tit, an idle-sounding bit of a bird. In winter, there's the smell of rain charged with woodsmoke — it's a town of fireplaces, with time to sit around them — and the sidewalks are strewn with the gray buttons of the eucalyptus' pods, and its sickle-shaped leaves.

This is our town as George in Washington must be remembering it. I suppose he wouldn't forget our 'characters' — the man who blows soap bubbles on the street corners for a lifework, or our town magician, or the tattered old wanderer who sticks fresh flowers all around his hatband every morning. Or the Franciscan monks, in sandals, robes, and Homburg hats.

Well, they're still here, George, but they're harder to see. No longer does the town belong to people sweetly doing nothing. Now suddenly the streets are flooded with living streams whose springs rise in every state of our Union. For to north of us and to the south are great army camps and giant naval bases; the boys in khaki, the boys in blue, the Marines in forest green have found us out — a town where they hope sweetly to do something, a furlough town, a liberty town, a town of old bells and young girls and open doors, full of people whose own sons, in uniform, are somewhere else.

The boys tell us they like our little city; so they came in a swelling river, and if you go about in the places where they are looking for fun, you get to know them. There goes that Arkansas boy whom we gave a lift to church the other day; there, sober now, goes the Tennessee marine who was asking for a buddy with a blacked eye; here's Sergeant Giuseppe Cimini from Assisi and Joysey City, who so earnestly will tell you that nobody born in this country can really appreciate it. There's that Minnesota lieutenant, operated on in the army hospital here last month, walking down the street with Heck's daughter.

Yes, you get to know a lot of them, and their names; you've been shown the pictures inside their wallets, maybe, even letters from home. More of them are nameless for you, but you won't forget them. Like migrant birds that depart, unnoticed because more come after them, they are going, gone. It's supposed to be a military secret where they are headed, after coming to the edge of the Pacific all the way from Boston or Savannah. And indeed it is a mystery, older than Egypt, where many of them will be voyaging. If God knows, He has not told it even to chiefs of staff.

It might strike an earnest spirit that all these boys from your town, out with these girls from mine, are pretty unreflecting and light-hearted, where they might stand awed on the blue brink of the Pacific. Indeed, when the clock's two hands creep up toward zenith, when the amber light in the bars grows blue and hazy, and over the juke-box tunes the voices rise louder and the laughter gets headier, a sober soul — if such be found there — might shake his head. That's when the sailors on liberty begin to be sure of the light little girls they have with them; that's when the flyers who are trying to make the young widow of one of their pals forget for a little, begin to succeed and themselves can relax. Yes, it's noisy; it sounds so gay that a strict moralist might well have reason to shake his head doubtfully. But if they are gay, it is because none of them can be really happy. Except for the strange, grave happiness that the best of them will sometimes, rarely, confide to you — the white peace at the center of a man who, loving life, is still willing to die, sure of what he may die for.

So, George, the platform on which you stood for Congress still stands here. The boys and girls are dancing on it, some their very last dance. There's going to be plenty of stamping, too, to shake it. But it's the only platform that will stand up under us all.

I've said that there were three great movements in American history: our westward push, our democratic revolution, our melting of many races into one nation. We are beginning to be conscious of a fourth. It is the movement in which those service men are marching toward the future. It is an expansion greater than our conquest of the West, a revolution greater than the complete democratizing of this one country of ours, a commingling into a vaster brotherhood than even America's. This fourth and most titanic movement in our history is that which convulses the world, but because of the standard we raised when we raised this nation, we cannot escape a leader's rôle in it. For we are the people who declared that all men are created equal. We are the land of the free, and we are now beginning to see that, in the words of Emporia's wise man, 'Liberty is the one thing you can't have unless you give it to others.' So that this forward surge in our national life comes from a newly realized obligation to the world outside ourselves. We were told at the beginning that we'd have to hang together or hang separately. We'd better believe it now.

As I look back through the long perspective of fallen leaves, into our past, I see the debating of those two men under an Illinois autumn sky as the first stir and struggle of this movement of responsibility. Not only was Lincoln calling upon his fellow citizens to feel responsible for their black brothers, but he announced then — and we'd better listen to it now — that a house divided against itself cannot stand. For the Abolitionists of New England were calling for disunion as loudly as the fire-eating Secessionists in Carolina. 'The Constitution of the United States is a covenant with death,' said orator Wendell Phillips of Boston. The Union, said others, was a compact with the devil. There were plenty more who wanted peace at any price. 'Let the Southern sisters depart in peace,' said many a Northern editor. And the South asked: 'Yes, why don't you let us? We only ask to be let alone. We would be friends with you, sharing glorious memories of the Revolution together, if you would but give us the right we both then fought for, the right of political independence, of self-determination.'

It sounds reasonable, just, and moderate. The conservative party always sounds so. The revolutionary party always sounds insistent and intransigent. The North took two stands, the one often disclaimed by the supporters of the other: the first, most keenly felt in the Northeast, was on the abolition of slavery, based on the assertion, to use Lincoln's words, that a man cannot be required to stand idle and see a second enslave a third. The other point of view was that the Union must be preserved, the house must not fall divided; this last was primarily the Middlewestern stand.

Never before, I think, had any people fought a long and terrible war for the privilege of remaining united with brothers who wished to depart from them. So utterly did they uphold this purpose that they preferred to be united in their graves at Shiloh and the Wilderness and Antietam and Chickamauga, rather than live in a peace estranged. It was a new kind of war, fought against brothers for brotherhood, though not all men saw it so at the time, or even afterward. But, if there must still be wars, it were best that they be fought for this ideal, and for the abolition of any persisting forms of slavery.

It is just as clear that in the South too men were fighting on different issues. Robert E. Lee did not own any slaves; I have never heard that he said a word in defense of slavery. The rank and file of Confederate soldiers owned no negroes. Out of a population of nine million people it is estimated that only about three hundred thousand had property rights in even one black man. Every black slave was the economic enemy of free white labor. And so, though the slave-owners made noisy demonstration, it is hardly conceivable that twenty-nine people would risk their lives and their fortunes to defend the property and theories of a thirtieth.

Suppose we say that the South was fighting for states' rights. If so, they had good historical ground for this stand; the Union had been entered into by sovereign and independent states; the Constitution was ambiguous on just how much power the states had delegated to the Federal Government, and just how much right they had to independence and secession. As an example, when the United States Supreme Court handed down the decision in the case of Chisholm *vs.* Georgia, giving an individual a right to sue a state, the state legislature of Georgia proposed an act declaring that anyone who tried to force a judgment based on this decision should be hanged. The measure didn't pass on a vote, but it showed a temper exhibited in one state after another to regard the federal authority as weaker than state authority. Such extreme views were not held by the majority of Southerners; to many of them the Union was a sanctified bond. Lee wrote his son, 'I can contemplate no greater calamity for the country than a dissolution of the Union.' Yet, when on the eve of conflict he was offered the command of the Union armies, he, a West Point graduate, sorrowfully declined. He could not, he said, draw his sword against his relatives and neighbors — a piece of reasoning perfectly comprehensible to a Virginian.

Not a slave-owner, a most reluctant secessionist, this fearless, noble, kind, and upright man was defending, with all the force of military genius and pure motive — what, then? 'A way of life,' I've heard it said. And perhaps this is the best explanation, although the North was not consciously attacking that way. It was a beautiful way, in some respects the fairest that America has produced from her soil. But it was not the way that the world was going. It was the last flower of the eighteenth century. And now the north wind had begun to tear at the petals.

The causes of a war have to be kept distinct in our minds from the reason that men go into the army, and both of these are separate from the ways that wars get started. If you ask why the rank and file, who were not interested in slavery one way or the other and couldn't define states' rights, went so gallantly to the Civil War, you get an age-old answer that fills the heart with pride and sorrow. Said Johnny Chestnut of Mississippi, 'No use to give a reason — a fellow could not stay away from the fight — not very well.'

All the world has heard that the Civil War started when the first shell went screaming up from the East Battery in Charleston over the silvery bay toward Fort Sumter. Who fired the shot and who ordered it? It's worth asking, because Major Anderson, in command of the fort, was a Southern sympathizer who had sent word to the Confederate forces that, as he soon would be starved out, they could have the place without a blow, if they would wait. Up in Richmond, Toombs, the Confederate Secretary of State, told Jefferson Davis, 'The firing upon that fort will inaugurate a civil war greater than any the world has yet seen. Mr. President, at this time it is suicide. ... You will wantonly strike a hornet's nest.... It is unnecessary; it puts us in the wrong: it is fatal.'

But others in power could not wait for the 'irrepressible conflict' to begin. The telegraph flashed the order to Charleston, and to Edwin Ruffin, as the oldest fire-eater present, was accorded the honor of setting off the first cannon. When Lee surrendered at Appomattox, Ruffin was to walk out in his garden, of a beautiful April day, and fire the shot that penetrated his heart. Behind him he left his famous curse upon the North and all its works — unaware of the curse he put upon the South.

But in Charleston the steeples of its beautiful churches, St. Michael's, St. Philip's, St. John's, vibrated with joy when Sumter fell. The Honorable J. D. Pope, walking the city's storied streets while the bells drowned the songs of the mockers, saw that ornament of the bar, Mr. James Petigru, puffing along and stamping his cane.

'Where's the fire, Judge? Where's the fire?' Petigru demanded.

'Mr. Petigru, there is no fire. Those are joy bells, ringing in honor of secession.'

'I tell you there is a fire. They have this day set a blazing torch to the temple of constitutional liberty, and we shall have no more peace forever.'

In St. Michael's Episcopal Church, the congregation held its breath as the minister prayed, 'O Lord, our heavenly Father, the high and mighty ruler of the Universe, who dost from thy throne behold all the dwellers upon earth, most heartily we beseech thee with thy favor to behold and bless thy servant the President of the Confederate States —' A soft, churchly hum, a sigh of relief and pride, breathed over all the congregation. But one handsome old citizen with a shock of unruly white hair and a heavy cane arose from his place, stepped into the aisle, turned his back upon the altar and with simple dignity, his eyes unflinching from the stares of his neighbors, walked out into the fragrant sunlight. His neighbors summed it up this way, afterward: 'South Carolina seceded from the Union. Jim Petigru stayed in it.'

And now the awful wave of war drew back in order to gather itself up, rise, tower, and surge forward, drowning and destructive. Now no man could stand against that surge; everyone in the nation was swept off his feet. Thirty million people struggled in that tidal current, were flung this way and that, fighting and strangling, sucked down to death, tossed up to heroism. Today the hatreds of the Civil War are dead; the wounds are closed; there is mutual forgiveness, and we have pride in each other's nerve and pluck. Over James Petigru's grave in St. Michael's yard rises the monument on which his fellow citizens have carved it deep that

> In the great Civil War
> He withstood his People for his Country:
> But his People did Homage to the Man
> Who held his Conscience higher than their Praise.

Once more, Americans have got through. We call it all an old story now, and that's the best way to think of it. But what a story! What an epic — American style, to be chanted to a banjo and sung around a campfire! There's a whole manner of music that any of us recognizes, from a single fragment of melody, as Civil War. The songs sound as though they ought naturally to go in the minor mode, but the singer is keeping them major. And when the boys in blue sang, 'Many the hearts that are weary tonight, wishing for the war to cease,' they were singing for both sides. Sometimes the two armies played concerts to each other, the Rappahannock running between them.

> Down flocked the soldiers to the banks,
> Till, margined by its pebbles,
> One wooded shore was blue with 'Yanks,'
> And one was gray with 'Rebels.'

Even about old newspaper verse with yellowed edges, there is still a whiff of powder. Even about a few plunked notes of 'The Land of Jubilo' there is a heartbeat that can still send a little blood breaking through the old wounds.

But only one great poet spoke for the Civil War; one singer lifts his voice above the touching sectional melodies. He wrote a sort of unholy Bible in which one can find anything. Walt Whitman, though he followed the Union armies, might have been writing for either side when he describes 'Cavalry Crossing a Ford,' 'Bivouac on a Mountainside,' 'A March in the Ranks Hard-Prest, and the Road Unknown,' 'As Toilsome I Wandered Virginia's Woods,' or this, which is as good today as when he wrote it:

Long, too long, America,
Traveling roads all even and peaceful you learn'd from joys and
 prosperity only,
But now, ah now, to learn from cries of anguish, advancing,
 grappling with direst fate and recoiling not,
And now to conceive and show to the world what your children
 en-masse really are.

But even Whitman, in the surging of the great wave, floundered and gasped and for the first eighteen months of the war was almost voiceless about it. The first Bull Run, Shiloh, Antietam, the second Bull Run were lost and won, and still the greatest American poet had not found his tongue, had not seen the front, had no personal stake acknowledged in the conflict. But Destiny had its eye on him nevertheless. For his brother, Captain George Whitman, was riding with Burnside's army toward Fredericksburg in Virginia. And now the wave is toppling above that little town.

It was a town foredoomed by geography, for it stands on a straight north-south line between Washington and Richmond, halfway between them, and just below the tiny city the Rappahannock widens out, a tidal stream difficult to cross. So Fredericksburg was pivot on the extreme right flank of Lee's line of defense, and on Burnside's extreme left. And the time had come to try to turn Lee's flank, all else having failed. So two hundred thousand young bodies are to be hurled into this little space together, with all the deathly cunning that brains can devise and all the courage that hearts can pump up. And the vultures begin to gather in the wintering skies above the little roofs, whence the swallows have departed.

There is a sort of terrible, mathematical simplicity about that battle. The lay of it can be described as easily as a map could do it. North of the Rappahannock is a line of hills, with the boys in blue on it. There is a fine old mansion on the height there, called Chatham, belonging to Major Lacy, who is over on the other side of the river fighting with the Confederates. In this house, where George and Martha Washington spent some nights of their honeymoon, every President — according to legend — had at some time been entertained; Lincoln had been here, not long before the battle, to review the troops, and under Chatham's old trees Robert E. Lee had courted the sweetheart he married. Down below flows the river, past Ferry Farm, peacefully along toward tidal waters. The bridges, of course, are blown up. And on the town shore, the buildings on the bank are filled with sharpshooters. The town itself, with its straight streets, its old trees and old churches and welcoming doorways, stands on a little shelf above the river. Behind the town, to the south of it, there was then an open field, with Queen-Anne's-lace and meadow-larks, in season, and above the field a hill. They call it Marye's Heights, and on the summit is the Marye house, white-porticoed and as gracious, in its own way, as Chatham.

On this hill Lee had drawn up his army; he had massed his artillery so that, in the words of a Confederate soldier, 'a chicken could not live upon that slope.' Grimly Lee and Longstreet and Stonewall Jackson waited for the great assault.

The battle began with a terrific artillery duel. All through the night of December 11 the black sky was opened with tongues of flame. Trees in the town were cut off at the stump; shells burst through the roofs of the houses, setting them afire, tumbling bed and table, china and silverware upon the terrified families in the cellars. As the Fredericksburgers fled next day before the holocaust, the Federal troops tried to build pontoons to cross the river, but when they were more than halfway across, the Confederate sharpshooters mowed down the engineers. At four o'clock in the afternoon not one bridge had been completed, and the engineers declared it impossible to go on.

Then the Federal officers called for volunteers to get into the pontoon boats and row them across under enemy fire. Two New York regiments, and the Seventh and Second Michigan, attempted the crossing. Under withering fire they poled their boats across; one half of them were killed before they reached the bank, but the rest rushed up and drove back the sharpshooters of Barksdale's Mississippi Brigade. The pontoons were laid, and the whole Federal army crossed over into the town.

For many a year the Michigan Second (my grandfather among them, and wounded that day) and the Michigan Seventh sang these words, to the melody of *Maryland, My Maryland*:

> Dark rolls the Rappahannock's flood,
> Michigan, my Michigan,
> The tide is crimson with our blood,
> Michigan, my Michigan.
> Although for us the day was lost,
> Yet it shall be our proudest boast
> At Fredericksburg the Seventh crossed,
> Michigan, my Michigan.

Michigan, green Michigan, young then and raw, uncouth and brave, this is a long way you have come from the farms with the red barns, from the dusty courthouse squares and the mustering ground among the burr oaks, where the flags hung limp in the hot August days. Hung curled so the stripes were tangled and the stars were lost in the folds. It is a long way to come from the northwoods and the loon lakes and the skyline pricked with spruce tops. What would you boys be doing, in the streets of this innocent little city? Why are you here, unwelcome, in the town where Washington grew up, where young Monroe practiced law, where John Paul Jones clerked in his brother's tailoring shop? Why are you marching between the hedges of box with its odor noble and serene, that has grown so much taller since it was planted?

We are here to carry the flag till it streams out straight again, till the stripes are uncrossed and the stars shine out once more from the midnight folds.

On the luckless 13th of December, in 1862, Burnside ordered an assault upon Marye's Heights. I do not know why generals do these things. We are told, correctly, that no layman can understand a battle, and it seems, from the many accounts I have read of this one, that few soldiers understood it either. One and all they had to read about it in the official reports afterward — those who survived — to find out what had happened. Burnside's staff deplored the assault beforehand, yet because their commander, under public pressure for a victory, demanded it, they had to send the boys they knew so well against a foe they knew well also.

The open slope up which they must charge was bad enough. But hidden from sight, halfway up it, there was a sunken road with a stone wall along it, forming a natural breastwork, behind which the Confederates had posted sharpshooters. Wave after wave of courage and youth broke on that wall. Watching from the tower of the Fredericksburg courthouse, General Couch saw what was happening to his regiments, saw them lean against the level hail of lead until they got within two hundred and fifty yards of the cannon mouths. 'My God, I never saw such fighting!' he said. 'See how our men, our poor fellows are falling. It is only murder now.'

'Six times did the enemy,' Lee wrote, 'press on with great determination.' If courage could have won, said Longstreet, the enemy would have won this day.

Hancock led a charge of five thousand veterans, and lost two out of every five. The sunken road was piled high, and still they came on. Humphreys took forward forty-five hundred who had never been in a battle before; with fixed bayonets they advanced to the very muzzles behind the stone wall. In one moment a thousand had fallen. Yet they wheeled in order, when the trumpet sounded a retreat, and marched back singing and hurrahing. The Army of the Potomac, in the battle of Fredericksburg, lost in casualties over an eleventh of its total force.

Over at Chatham, Burnside was mad with grief. He wanted to put himself at the head of his old corps and lead a charge in which he hoped to die or redeem his honor. But his officers restrained him. Out on the battlefield an icy rain began to fall.

20

'Flag of Stars'

UPON THE DARKENING battlefield at Fredericksburg, his right arm mangled, lay a boy not long out of school. If he had any hopes of survival, they were that the enemy stretcher-bearers might find him; then, if he lived that long, he would meet the surgeon's knife dripping bacterial filth. After that, if he escaped gangrene, he would be transferred to a Confederate prison camp, there to battle typhoid, typhus, pneumonia, and tuberculosis. As he lay on the field of agony, the best he could hope to see was the old yellow hospital flag coming, with its associations of quarantine and death. For in 1862 no one had yet looked upon the blood-bright emblem of the Red Cross.

A woman's face appeared above him, a human angel with dark compassionate eyes, long tender mouth, and hands like his mother's. Save his own mother there was no person in the world he would have been so glad to see. For he recognized his old teacher, Miss Barton, Clara Barton of the low, sweet voice, who had never punished a child, in an age of plentiful school thrashings; Miss Barton who by sheer comradeship had conquered the hobbledehoy toughs taller than she. Clara Barton, whom everybody loved.

With a sob the boy flung his left arm around her neck, and buried his face in the cloak of the pitying woman. 'Do you know me?' he cried. 'I am Charley Hamilton, who used to carry your satchel home from school!' Charley's right arm, she saw, would never carry a satchel again.

At Clara Barton's call, stretcher-bearers came for Charley. Across the field a surgeon's lantern wavered toward them. There was just one woman on that field, and hundreds of men needed her.

So this little woman — she was exactly five feet tall and forty years of age, slender, nervous, almost morbidly responsive to suffering — daily and hourly met with her womanhood the man-made agonies of war. She was great enough for the encounter. In Civil War times no mere lady even dreamed of nursing at the front; husband-hunting ninnies were turned back every day. The army nurses, who had to qualify first through personal selection by aged and overworked Dorothea Dix, seldom left the walls of the base hospitals, where only a small fraction of the wounded ever arrived.

Clara Barton, the future founder of the American Red Cross, went out on the field. She belonged to no organization, had no official standing, and reached the desperately wounded only by battling for passes through the naturally preoccupied resistance of generals, surgeons, the Sanitary Commission, quartermasters, and supply-train drivers. She was simply a compassionate woman who, sometimes assisted by a few other women, sometimes hindered even by her friends, fought the pitched battle of mercy against Mars.

Clara Barton was born near Worcester, Massachusetts, in 1821, on Christmas Day. To me it seems that she was one of the few persons in the history of the human race not miserably unworthy of the comparison which that anniversary invites.

From her father, an old Indian-fighter, she had gained a precocious mastery of military affairs. She knew a major from a colonel when she could hardly see his uniform for mud or darkness; she remembered regimental numbers, listened without a blush to the blue swearing of army muleteers beside her on the wagon trains, and she comprehended the respective duties of the Sanitary Commission, the army surgeon, and the quartermaster. Unlike most women in wartime, she never considered herself an exception to the rule; she went where she was told, and troubled to obtain the right sort of passport. Military men quickly came to perceive all this; regiments recognized her, and cheered her as she trudged past them in the rain, going up to the front with clothes, bandages, fruits, jellies, sweets, wines, messages from home.

It was after the first battle of Bull Run that Clara Barton, then a clerk in the Patent Office at the capital, had begun to realize that every hour that elapses between a wound and arrival at a base hospital increases in geometrical ratio the likelihood of death. Men who might have been saved if their forces had been rallied at the start were hopeless cases before they reached the operating tents. She saw men who had been waiting so long in the stretcher queues that their feet had rotted off from gangrene, and she fought that fatal delay.

Surgeons sometimes opposed her. Regulation army nurses often looked coldly upon her. But Clara Barton knew that Ladies' Aid Societies at home were not enough, nor was the Sanitary Commission, and by sheer force of accomplishment slowly she won her way. When a doctor shaking with fatigue staggered from the operating tent where his last candle had guttered out, through the darkness a small cloaked figure came toward him, behind her a man bearing a whole chest of candles. When the anesthetics gave out, Clara Barton was there with stimulants. She soon learned that 'missing' was the most ominous word in the ghastly reports of the battles. She found thousands of missing men for their families.

Behind her she had only two slim organizations, a group of women in Worcester and another in Bordentown, New Jersey — little towns, that's all, but with big-hearted people in them. They helped, and Clara Barton used her own money without thought. For herself, dainty and feminine though she was, she spent practically nothing, like a nun, a lay Sister of Charity. In spite of the opposition of Secretary of War Stanton, she found army friends who helped her; they would tell her when a big battle was coming on. 'Follow the cannon' was her motto. And when the soldiers saw her, they joked, 'Here comes the stormy petrel!'

At Fredericksburg, with the troops, she crossed the Rappahannock under that murderous fire, ahead of all the army doctors and nurses. In the streets a man to whom she stopped to give a drink was shot dead in her arms; the bullet went through her sleeve. It was a rent she never mended.

At Chatham, those days after the battle, the stormy petrel — in truth a dark dove of mercy — found that 'twelve hundred men were crowded into the Lacy House, which contained but twelve rooms. They covered every foot of the floors and porticoes and even lay on the stair landings!' Through that crowd, unknown to each other, moved Clara Barton and Walt Whitman, who had come to seek his brother the captain. The man with the brushy beard and rubicund face, with the sombrero cocked over a heavy-lidded, pitying, and too knowing eye, must have remarked the quick, prim, trim woman with the bit of red at her throat. Miss Barton had a passion for red; there was always a fleck of it about her frugal dress. Though it had not yet taken the shape of a cross, it seemed to symbolize for her the heart's blood which she put into her work. She saw Walt, no doubt, but her business was with the broken and dying; as for him, he found his brother, wounded, but now he found too that these were all his brothers. Those walls echoed with agony, and outside, Walt writes, 'I notice a heap of amputated feet, legs, arms, hands, etc., about a load for a one-horse cart.' Into that vintage trampled from the grapes of wrath, two of the amplest souls our nation ever bore distilled a Godlike love that sanctifies the wine.

They went their separate ways, he to walk the base hospitals in Washington as a lay father confessor, and she to follow the cannon. Fredericksburg, shattered, burned, looted, was to change hands seven times in the Civil War. Chancellorsville, the Wilderness, and Spottsylvania remembered for the 'bloody angle' — they were all fought within cannon sound of this little town of my love. When at last the cannon had gone wheeling and thundering south and east, on the great three-quarters circle that was to end at Appomattox, the town knew peace again, the sort of peace that comes when you see daylight after a night of horror. Time has sweetened that; a tired old beauty is restored to the place and, when winter breaks, the hyacinths and squills come up in the dooryards as jauntily as ever. But today there are soldiers in the streets again, and Marines from Quantico. One of these, who fathered my godson, writes me he has just found a two-hundred-year-old house there, a Washington family house, in which to live a few intense week-ends with his young wife and the baby he scarcely knows. So the old heart of that town beats, as always, with the throb of love and glory; it is touched by destiny; it cannot forget what it knows.

> Listen! Again the shrill-lipped bugles blow
> Where the swift currents of the river flow
> Past Fredericksburg.

One of those trumpets, my old friend and neighbor Tom Ripley proudly tells me, is preserved in the G.A.R. rooms in his home town of Rutland, Vermont. I haven't seen that trumpet that sounded the charge of Fredericksburg, but Tom has put in my palm for a moment the Congressional Medal awarded his father for gallantry at Malvern Hill. Last spring, coming up through Virginia in dogwood time, I stopped the car all of a sudden because in those quiet woods there was a small roadside sign saying 'Malvern Hill.' It was startling to come upon it, for my mind was not on the Civil War; I had just been visiting the colonial splendors of Williamsburg; I had stopped at William Byrd's mansion of Westover and, a mile or two beyond it (such is the cosy propinquity of Virginia's heroic cradles), at the old Harrison place. Leisurely rolling along, we had crossed the honeymoon trail of Thomas and Martha Jefferson, and both of us were still aglow with old tidewater glories. And then, among the innocent Judas trees and the pines, that sign, that memory. One more of Virginia's bleeding names that, like a sword stroke, cut every thread you follow in her history.

It's easy to see why Lee loved Virginia so much, why all Virginians love it, and how they could have come to think of it as a part that was greater than the whole. How beautiful it is, tidewater, piedmont, and mountains — harmonious chord! It is like a great mansion, generous and gracefully furnished, with rooms in it for lovers, for many children, for the honored old. But in America's house are many mansions.

Their names make a poem, however you say them. Names of queen states, Maryland, Virginia, Carolina, names like flowers carried between smiling lips, Florida, California. Names thrust like eagle feathers in a big brave's hair, Kentucky, Michigan, Iowa, Illinois. Or, dug out of aboriginal earth, names such as Utah and Nebraska and Kansas, old arrowheads to keep for luck in the pocket. And then the one name, that Tom Paine found — the United States of America.

So no part is greater than the whole. To believe that it can be is the essential fallacy. No state on earth can be so sovereign that it stands above consideration of the interests of others. This planet is the mansion of the human race. To set that house in order must be what we are fighting for; doubt that it can be done breaks faith with all our past which has flowered in so nearly perfect a union. Among the nations we are Fortune's heir, and with great fortune comes responsibility. To accept it is to kneel for the crown of true sovereignty.

Pride married with humility bears a pure spirit, in any man, in any nation. I met that mood, the day before I set forth for my journey into America. It was the fairest and the darkest day I ever saw in Washington. It was the day of the fall of Bataan. The city was dressed for Easter, every fountain playing, every little flowering tree in blossom, all the great monuments shining against the dreamy background of Virginia hills. Not only did the uniforms of all our services, the flags of all the United Nations, make this the capital of the world, but some strong warm breath, some wind of spring's resurrecting passion, kept those flags whipped out streaming against clear blue sky.

I suppose, of all who have ever waited there, none were ever more awed than my wife and I, as we sat alone in the Green Room of the White House. The great busy mansion was very silent; the April day was so warm that an air-cooling unit was somewhere softly thrumming. It made you think of the engines at work deep in the heart of a mighty ship. And I thought, of this ship of state, that though the course must be dangerous, it is more dangerous still to hug the past like a worn shore full of well-known reefs. It is more dangerous to be small than great. It is safer to dare, it is richer to be open-handed, it is wiser to believe than to doubt.

I felt how the ship had taken a blow, this day, to make it shudder, and yet how unswervingly it kept to its course. Bataan, though the throat ached with thinking about it, was one with the battles that have been and have yet to be. Harrodsburg, Salinas, many another little town was hit to the heart, and in this place too the news brought a black hour, just as the news of Fredericksburg must have done.

They came, after that battle, generals, eye-witnesses, editors, politicians, and perhaps some of them waited in this room where I was sitting. And they told old Abraham what had happened. A mistake had been made — Lincoln's own, for appointing Burnside, Burnside's for overriding his officers, the public's mistake for asking a quick victory by strategy, by assault. The news of that mistake would go into every home, every little town, just in time for Christmas; in Marblehead whose volunteers had been the first to reach the mustering at Faneuil Hall, there would be more sorrow to add to the loss of her sailors who went down on the old wooden ship, the *Cumberland*, when the new ironclad *Merrimac* rammed her in Hampton Roads. Such was the price we were paying, in the last dark days of 'sixty-two, when Lincoln walked this house, when he wrote here past midnight, when he let himself out of the west wing and walked over to the War Department to ask for news at the telegraph table.

We sat in the Green Room, waiting, for five precise minutes by my watch; we had come five minutes early. We spoke a little, but softly, in appreciation of the tall dignity of this place, the crystal chandelier, the portraits on the walls. They were the longest five minutes I can ever remember, because they were so crowded with an overpowering sense of the history in this house. Here Thomas Jefferson had planned with his secretary, Meriwether Lewis, the expedition to the Pacific. Andrew Jackson, 'Old Hickory,' had shaken his stick at secession and stilled all talk of it. Grover Cleveland had defied the forces of greed that would have taken control of the government. Woodrow Wilson had foreshadowed the world as it must yet come to be. Like Lincoln, like Franklin Roosevelt, they all had their implacable enemies. There is a significant continuity about that enmity and its sources. There is a glorious continuity about all our great Presidents and their purpose.

The mind strained forward, trying to imagine the men who were to be Executive here. Though this country was again in deadly peril at this moment, one thing was certain: there would always be a President here, freely elected, representing the people. There would always come great ones, now and then, great in new ways no more possible to foresee than Washington could have foreseen Lincoln. But they could never outgrow the White House, so simple yet so lofty among the palaces of the world.

Wherever the mind went, in those minutes, exploring the house and remembering its occupants, Lincoln came oftenest to haunt it. There were fragments of his words in the air:

> It is for us the living, rather, to be dedicated here to the unfinished work which they who fought here have thus far so nobly advanced. It is rather for us to be here dedicated to the great task remaining before us — that from these honored dead we take increased devotion. . . .

With malice toward none, with charity for all, with firmness in the right as God gives us to see the right, let us strive on to finish the work we are in, to bind up the nation's wounds, to care for him who shall have borne the battle and for his widow and his orphan — to do all which may achieve and cherish a just and lasting peace among ourselves and with all nations.

In the doorway our names were spoken in summons, and we rose, as you are brought to your feet by the flag. It is going forward, that flag, in the hands of its standard bearer; we all see it waver, above the crowds and confusion, for a flag is a living thing, and trembles and flutters. But a great wind has caught its folds.

It is a new wind, and no man seems to know from what quarter it is blowing, or where it will carry our banner. It is not an east wind, nor a west wind; it's the wind of the world, of the planet's revolution.

Thick-sprinkled bunting! flag of stars!
Long yet your road, fateful flag — long yet your road, and lined
    with bloody death,
For the prize I see at issue at last is the world. . . .
O hasten, flag of man —
Flag of stars! Thick-sprinkled bunting!

THE END

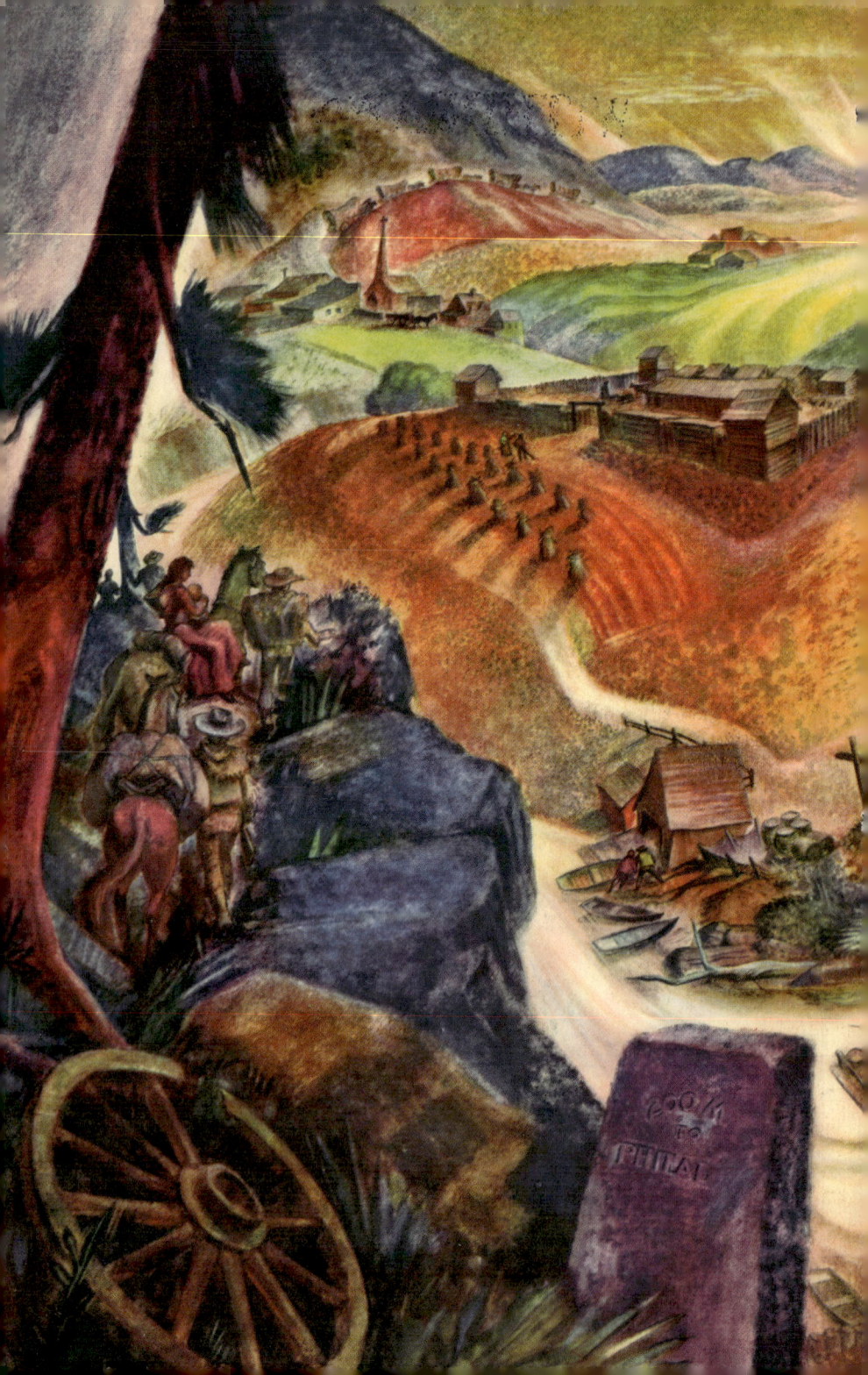